SPI
EGE
L&G
RAU

LIVING AND DYING IN BRICK CITY

LIVING AND DYING IN BRICK CITY

An E.R. Doctor Returns Home

SAMPSON DAVIS

with Lisa Frazier Page

Spiegel & Grau

New York

Copyright © 2013 by Sampson Davis

All rights reserved.

Published in the United States by Spiegel & Grau, an imprint of The Random House Publishing Group, a division of Random House, Inc., New York.

SPIEGEL & GRAU and design is a registered trademark of Random House, Inc.

LIBRARY OF CONGRESS CATALOGING-IN-PUBLICATION DATA

Davis, Sampson.

Living and dying in Brick City : an E.R. doctor returns home / Sampson Davis.

p.;cm.

Includes bibliographical references.

ISBN 978-1-4000-6994-1 (alk. paper) — ISBN 978-0-679-60518-8 (ebook)

I. Title.

[DNLM: 1. Davis, Sampson. 2. Physicians—New Jersey—Autobiography. 3. Emergency Medicine—New Jersey. 4. Internship and Residency—New Jersey. 5. Medically Underserved Area—New Jersey. 6. Urban Health Services—New Jersey. WZ 100]

610.92—dc23

[B]

2012029647

Printed in the United States of America on acid-free paper.

www.spiegelandgrau.com

2 4 6 8 9 7 5 3 1

First Edition

Book design by Chris Welch

Mom, this one is for you.
You were the first person to teach me the most
important ingredient in medicine: compassion.

CONTENTS

LIVING AND DYING IN BRICK CITY

INTRODUCTION

I t was just before 7:00 A.M. on July 1, 1999, my first full day on the job. Jay-Z blared from the stereo as I steered my old Honda Accord past the White Castle burger joint, toward Newark Beth Israel Medical Center. The neighborhood—a mix of boarded-up buildings, dingy brick storefronts, beauty supply stores, and fast-food restaurants—rolled by like a video. Before long, the July heat would draw residents out of their homes to play checkers and cards, children in swimsuits would be dashing through open fire hydrants, and sweaty boys would be swooshing basketballs through naked rims on concrete courts. This was Brick City, *my* city. I knew its rhythms, and I'd seen its dark side up close. Even at this time of morning, I could see glimpses of it: the homeless old man sleeping next to a junk-filled grocery cart and a couple of half-naked women still strutting the blocks from the night before. The dope boys and other hustlers would be out later, too, stirring up all kinds of trouble—trouble that at times has given my home-town a reputation as one of the most dangerous cities in America. I used to be one of those confused boys, a kid with potential I didn't even know existed inside of me, a kid who wanted better but for the longest time couldn't crystallize in my mind what that might look like, let alone how to get it. That seemed like a lifetime ago.

I slowed down to enter the zone around the hospital, one of New Jersey's premier medical institutions. Its sprawling redbrick buildings towered over both sides of Lyons Avenue and consumed practically the entire block. I turned into the five-story parking garage across from the hospital's main entrance and smiled at the funny ways of fate. Here I was, a doctor now, pulling in to the same hospital where eight years earlier, one summer evening after my senior year in high school, I'd spent practically the entire night parked outside the ambulance entrance with two carloads of my friends. We'd rushed to the hospital with a friend who was convinced that the marijuana he'd just smoked was about to kill him. But when we got there, we were too scared to go inside for help and too high to know better. We'd been drinking that hot summer night, and my friend had decided to try some weed for the first time. Then the buzz he'd anticipated didn't happen fast enough.

"Aww, Marshall, this ain't nothing," he'd said, calling me the middle name used by my family and old friends. "I can't get high."

He kept smoking and smoking. Then sweat started popping out all over his face, and his heart rate sped up. "Feels like it's about to beat outta my chest," he said, panting and pleading with us not to let him die.

We jumped in our cars and drove to Beth. Between cracking up with laughter and feeling scared out of our minds, we debated the consequences of going inside. Like me, my incapacitated friend was one of the few in our group headed to college. What would happen if the E.R. doctors discovered that he was not really about to die, but instead high? Would this go on some kind of record and get him kicked out of college before he even started?

"It's just the weed, man. It's just the weed," we told him repeatedly, trying to calm his fear that he was about to meet his maker. We came up with a plan: We'd sit with him in the car and pace with him on the street to give the weed time to wear off, but we'd stay parked outside the emergency room, in case. If our friend looked like he was about to pass out, we would only have to rush a few steps inside. My mom always said God looks out for babies and fools, and the good Lord must have been looking out for us that night. The weed wore off without my friend having a heart attack, and we got back in our cars and drove home. Who could have guessed then that old Marshall someday would have his own parking space in the doctors' lot at Beth?

I steered into one of the reserved spots on the first floor of the garage and stepped out of my car. I draped my stethoscope around my neck, pulled on my white lab coat, smoothed it back and front, then ran my hand over the black thread embroidered across the top left side: Sampson M. Davis, M.D., Emergency Medicine.

I liked the feel of it.

Through some miracle, I had not only survived these merciless streets but also ended up as a doctor at the same hospital where I took my first breath. Fresh out of medical school, I was now on the other side of the desperation and despair: the healing side. From this unique vantage point, I would come to see the community where I was raised and the high price of poverty in a whole new way. I would see lives that might have been saved if the industrious young men landing in my emergency room full of bullet holes had learned and believed that education offered a better alternative. I would see young women giving up their power and entrusting their health to unworthy men—and dying because of it. I would see health issues out of control—obesity, diabetes, heart disease, stroke—and behaviors that unwittingly perpetuated a disproportionate rate of death. And I would see myself.

There are plenty of books by doctors who have shared their experiences working in a hospital or their expertise on various health issues, but few have drawn attention to the health crisis in our inner cities. The violence, the despair, the poverty, the hopelessness—they all have been examined as societal, social, and cultural issues; yet there are inextricable medical issues as well. These are the physical and mental health conditions that play out night after night in emergency rooms across the country and sap communities of their strength and vitality. After more than a decade working on the front line of healthcare in my own beleaguered community, I have seen remarkable resilience, but I have also witnessed far too many tragedies. That is why I am sharing these stories, along with information that can mean the difference between illness and health, between life and death.

Some names and physical descriptions have been changed to protect the identities of those who have suffered and, in some cases, the families they left behind. But every story is real. My hope is that this book will inspire change. That it will open eyes wider to the serious health problems facing a too-often overlooked population. That it will encourage political and community leaders, medical professionals, and others with brilliant minds, creative ideas, and positions of influence to make a difference on this front. But most of all I hope that men and women living in the conditions described here will see themselves and their loved ones in these stories, turn away from self-destructive behaviors, and seek appropriate medical help.

For me, emergency medicine has been a calling, a vocation connected to my higher purpose. Ultimately, this book is part of that, another way to do what I got into medicine to do in the first place: help save lives.

1

BROTHERS

Brother, brother, brother
There's far too many of you dying. . . .
—*Marvin Gaye, 1971*

T he name stopped me cold.
Don Moses.
I knew a Don Moses. And I knew right away it had to be him.

I'd been in my residency for several months, but this was my first day on duty in the trauma unit at University Hospital, one of the training centers in Beth Israel's network. I'd made it to the conference room early for the morning report, coffee cup in hand, my green scrubs and white lab coat spotless. The least I could do was look polished. There would be lots of gray hair and experience in the room, and I'd heard that these sessions could be brutal. Word was, the senior surgeons often challenged the medical actions taken the night before by their less-experienced colleagues, and they didn't think twice about knocking an ill-prepared resident down to size. Fortunately for me, as a newbie I wasn't on the hot seat. My plan was to lie low, watch, and learn. But I couldn't take my eyes off the green chalkboard at the front of the room—and that name, in white chalk, crossed out, with a word written next to it in all caps: "DECEASED."

Don Moses.

It jumped out from the long list of patient names and data. The age seemed about right, thirty-one, just four years older than me. And he probably would have come to this hospital, since it was close to the old neighborhood. He'd been shot several times, had made it through surgery, and had been in the Surgical Intensive Care Unit. And then, that line through his name. My eyes froze there, my knees went weak, and I eased into my seat for the morning report. Suddenly, my cool began to melt. The cotton lab coat that I'd pulled on just moments earlier now felt like wool, and the once ice-cold conference room was starting to feel like a sauna.

Don Moses.

We called him Snake. A decade had passed since I'd seen him dashing past me with the police on his heels one wild summer night. I'd lived across the street from the eight-story Dayton Street projects, one of Newark's most notorious housing developments, and I hung out there practically every day. As a teenager, Snake had moved to the Seth Boyden projects, a short walk away. His fearless swagger and willingness to scrap with anybody who got in his way quickly earned him the respect of the toughest dudes around. The Dayton Street grammar school sat between the two housing projects, and from the time my friends and I were old enough to play outside alone, the schoolyard was our main hangout. We grew up playing hide-and-go-seek and shooting hoops there. Then, as teenagers, we'd sit on the concrete steps and pass the time listening to music, rapping, and talking about girls. I held a gun for the first time one summer night on that playground. I was seventeen. Snake, Duke, Manny, and I took turns passing around the cold, hard steel. It was Duke's gun; he'd bought it off some kid on the street. Duke was the one who'd introduced us to Snake. Both were in their early twenties. The night Duke brought the gun to the yard, he and Snake took practice shots into the school's metal door. Holding the nine-millimeter pistol was enough excitement for me. It just didn't feel right blasting bullets through a schoolhouse door. But that night sealed our bond. The four of us became a team, with Manny and me as the eager-to-please little brothers.

We looked up to Snake. He was a mysterious dude, about five feet ten inches tall and two hundred pounds of solid muscle. He was smooth on his feet, although he moved through the neighborhood with a huge walking stick. His friends knew its real purpose: It would double as a whipping stick for the fools who dared to try to catch him off guard. He usually wore baseball caps to cover a patch of missing hair from a permanent scalp injury, which probably happened during a street fight. Snake was always down to fight. But his allegiance was flighty at best. He'd scrap one-on-one against a neighborhood rival or battle with a group targeting another gang. But he'd sometimes do an about-face and attack guys I thought were his boys. You never knew what to expect from Snake or how far he would go. During battle, the dude seemed to have no emotions; he'd beat an opponent mercilessly, past the point where even a little bit of human empathy might have said, "That's enough." In that sense, he was a real warrior, and back then it felt good to be on Snake's side. There was a fun part of him, too. He was the first to pull a prank or talk music and girls, but even then he never revealed much about himself. I sometimes saw him with his sister, but he never talked about his family or home life.

I don't know whether Snake ever finished high school, but neither he nor Duke worked a real nine-to-five; they mostly hustled drugs and did odd jobs to keep cash and make themselves appear legitimate. The summer before my senior year in high school, the four of us were hanging out in the schoolyard one night as usual, when Duke came up with a moneymaking scheme to rob drug dealers. I knew it was wrong, but we wouldn't be hurting anybody, I reasoned. They were just drug dealers. And something about the idea made me feel powerful and strong. At fifteen, Manny already had some prior arrests; he was game right away. Part of me was becoming as comfortable as my friends with this thug life, but there was another side of me, too.

As quiet as I'd kept it, I was also an honor student at University High School, where I'd become best friends with two other guys, Rameck and George. We'd ended up in some of the same classes and clicked right away because all three of us did well in school and still managed to be popular and cool. At the end of the previous school year, our junior year, George had talked Rameck and me into applying together to a scholarship program that would provide almost a full ride to college *and* medical school if we wanted to become doctors. None of us could have afforded college otherwise (even if the medical school part still seemed iffy for me), and so we'd taken the leap, sure of just one thing: Whatever we didn't know we could figure out together. I hadn't dared to mention any of those plans to Snake and the boys, though. They would have laughed me off the stoop: Marshall, going to college? Becoming a doctor? Who did I think I was? Some rich white dude or one of those Cosby kids on TV? Around my way, it was all about the here and now. Tomorrow wasn't promised, and you did what you had to do today to survive.

For the moment, robbing drug dealers was the plan. What happened next seemed part of some bad dream—from us jumping out one night on the young Montclair drug boys to Snake and Duke brandishing the firepower to my patting down pockets and snatching jewelry and cash. All four of us had dressed in black to blend in with the darkness. We were just about to make our getaway when I noticed a brown four-door Chevy Citation pull up to the curb on the street in front of us. Two men in jeans and polo shirts shouted some questions about being lost. I moved discreetly toward the car and noticed a police radio on the floor. I immediately began backing away from the scene, yelling: "21 Jump! 21 Jump!" Undercover cops. We'd taken the code from the name of a popular television series.

Within seconds, we were practically surrounded by police cars. My ten-second jump-start helped me distance myself from the scene and appear more like a spectator. The police focused on my three friends. As Snake sprinted past me, his sweaty face glistening, his gold chain bouncing on his chest, he looked shocked and desperate. It had never occurred to us that we might get caught. *Keep your head straight, Sam,* I told myself. *Keep walking. Don't run just yet. Blend in with the surroundings. You're seconds away from freedom.*

All three of my boys were arrested that night, and their loyalty ended there. Police found my ride, the would-be getaway car, at the scene and put out the word that they were coming for me. I turned myself in the next day. Because of their ages, Snake and Duke were taken to jail. Manny and I were transported to a juvenile detention center. To this day, I thank God that I was only seventeen and a half. If this had occurred a few months later, my future would have been a very different story. Since all three had serious priors, Snake was sentenced to seven years, Duke got five years, and Manny four. With just a misdemeanor shoplifting charge to my name, I got probation and, after four weeks in juvenile detention, another chance.

That experience changed me. I wasn't familiar enough with the world outside Dayton Street to know for sure what I wanted out of life, but after my time in juvenile detention, I realized jail wasn't it. All of the warnings from my parents, teachers, and others suddenly had become real. *Never again,* I told myself. Never again would I spend a night sleeping behind bars on a razor-thin cot that smelled like piss. Never again would I have to listen to dudes being raped while constantly watching my own back. Never again would I look into my mother's eyes and see the pain and disappointment that I'd put there. When I got out, I returned to University High for my senior year and started hanging out more with Rameck and George.

I was playing basketball at the schoolyard one day during my probation when I ran into Snake and Duke. They were out on bail and hadn't been sentenced yet. We shot hoops together for a while like we used to and tried hanging out in our old spot, but it was too uncomfortable. None of us mentioned our arrests, but the air was tense. They probably had heard I'd received probation and resented that I wouldn't have to do serious time. We didn't have much to say to each other. Things were clearly different. I was different, and I knew then that the friendship was over. I never saw Snake again. I later heard that as soon as he got out of jail, he returned to the streets. And then I hadn't heard or seen his name for years—until now.

The half hour in the conference room zipped by in a blur. As soon as it ended, I asked a colleague to point the way to the Surgical Intensive Care Unit and ran down the hall in search of the room number that had been listed next to Snake's real name on the board. I rounded the corner and noticed a small group of people gathered in the hall outside the room. Some were crying. A few of the faces looked vaguely familiar. When one of the women glanced up at me, my heart stopped. The lump in my throat felt like a boulder. It was Snake's sister. I could see in her red, puffy eyes that she recognized me, too. What was she thinking? Did she resent me because I hadn't gotten jail time like her brother had? Guilt washed over me, and I felt a sudden urge to explain. I wanted to tell her that I'd needed to let her brother go to find my own way. The family members' eyes followed me. I could hear their voices inside my head: *Wasn't he the one who used to hang out with Snake? Who does he think he is, coming here now? He thinks he's so special.* I wanted to pull up a chair, grieve with them, and assure them that it was me, the same old Marshall. I wanted to show them that I hadn't abandoned Snake, that I hadn't abandoned them, that if I hadn't made new friends, if I hadn't gone to college, I would have ended up here, too, right beside Snake. As I ambled up to Snake's sister, I realized that I never even knew her name. I fumbled for the right words.

"I'm sorry," I said.

Snake's sister nodded kindly. He had died the night before, she confirmed. I wondered for a moment whether I should hug her, but it felt too awkward. I asked her to pass along my condolences to the rest of the family, and I excused myself. I slipped past the crowd and into the room where Snake had been. It was empty and a bit eerie. The covers on Bed 6, where he once lay, were still pulled back, and a host of medical machines—ventilator, cardiac monitor, IV pump—sat motionless. Snake's body had been taken to the morgue, but I still stood there in silence, looking around the room, thinking, *This so easily could have been me.*

The swell of emotions was confusing: pain, regret, gratitude, guilt. I remembered Snake's cool laugh, his witty remarks, his collection of baseball caps. I wondered if beneath all that bravado and rage he'd had dreams, like me, but had been too afraid to share them, or whether life had choked every bit of hope from him from the start. I wondered if I could have said something that might have made a difference. I wondered about all the things I never even knew or thought to ask him—what his mother was like, whether his father was part of his life, whether he'd ever had a teacher or counselor who'd told him he was smart. Kids aren't born without hope. But it's easy to grow up where we grew up, seeing death and destruction around us all the time, and think it's normal. And it's also difficult to hope for a life you've never seen beyond the television screen, to believe it is truly within your grasp.

Like a survivor pulled from the wreckage over a pile of dead bodies, I stood in that hospital room wondering: *Why? Why me? Why had I survived? Why had I made it out?* The guilt felt so overwhelming that I couldn't think clearly.

The brothers kept coming. Night after night. Week after week. Young men, wasting their skills and smarts on the streets, young brothers who reminded me of the person I used to be. Then came one whose physical appearance made me do a double take.

It was an uncharacteristically hot day in April 2001 when I heard a commotion in the ambulance entrance outside the hospital.

"We need a stretcher over here!" a security guard yelled.

He was the first to notice the guy who had somehow lifted himself from a nearby sidewalk and stumbled around the corner to the glass doors of the ambulance bay. He was pounding on the door with the little energy he had left. His bloody hand streaked the clear glass a dark red.

"We need help now!" the guard persisted.

I grabbed the first free stretcher I saw and dashed with other hospital workers toward the noise. Outside, the patient I would come to know as Legend lay slumped against the door. His tattered flesh oozed blood from quarter-sized holes all over his body. We lifted him onto the gurney and ran at top speed toward the resuscitation bay. I was glad I'd worn my Nike sneakers with my scrubs that day. Comfort was important, and so was the ability to move fast.

"Doc, I'm going to die," Legend uttered, spitting up blood. He was determined to get the words out: "Please tell my family, my kids, I love them."

I looked down to reassure him and was startled by what I saw: His face resembled mine. Legend appeared to be in his late twenties, like me, with the same muscular medium build, the same honey-colored complexion, and the same neat, short haircut. He seemed dazed, and his eyes followed my every move. He reached up for my hand and attempted to speak. Instead, more blood spurted out.

"Hang in there, man," I said. "You are not going to die."

But who was I fooling? The more clothes we cut off, the more bullet holes I counted. Legend had taken two gun blasts to the abdomen, another two to the chest, and there were two superficial wounds. The high-caliber bullets had torn through his vital organs. The floor in the trauma bay was now slippery with his blood, and I struggled to keep my footing as I maneuvered quickly around the bed and hooked him to a heart monitor. His blood pressure was low and his heart rate high. Another member of the team inserted an IV to deliver a saline solution and blood. He was struggling for air, so I hurriedly inserted a breathing tube in his mouth to connect him to a ventilator. With obvious bullet wounds in the chest and trouble breathing, he most likely had a collapsed lung. I needed to insert a chest tube, and quickly. I'd done it only twice before, but I knew better than to hesitate. My years of street sports always helped me through tricky times like these. Back then I'd had the confidence I needed to go for the winning shot in pickup basketball. I talked myself into that same zone now as I grabbed a scalpel and made a two-inch incision on the side of his chest: *You've got this. You can do it. Stay calm and steady.*

Next, I probed the cavity with a blunt instrument, trying to make my way to the lung. It took only a few seconds to puncture the connective tissue and reach it. A whoosh of air and then a rush of blood spurted out of the hole. The lung had collapsed and looked like a crumpled wad of paper. As the built-up pressure inside the chest cavity escaped, the shriveled lung began to reexpand. I placed the chest tube, which looked like a small garden hose, into the chest cavity and hooked it to the vacuum. The reinflated lung adhered to the inner chest wall, as it should have, giving Legend more time. But blood was pouring into the tube quicker than the vacuum could suction it out.

In a last-ditch effort to save his life, we cracked open his chest to see if we could close a hole in or near the heart by clamping off damaged blood vessels, but when we reached the heart, we discovered that there was no more blood. All four chambers were empty. There was nothing more we could do. *Damn!* I snapped off my bloody plastic gloves, took a moment to steady myself, and headed for the waiting room. The look on my face must have spoken before I said even a word. Legend's mother screamed for God and fell to her knees. A clump of hospital workers gathered around to comfort her. That's when I realized she was a hospital employee herself, part of the Beth Israel family. This kind of news, never easy to deliver, was even tougher now. "I'm sorry," I said. "We did everything we could." Legend's mother was inconsolable. A crowd of about fifty people kept vigil outside the hospital. They stood around the ambulance bay in tight clusters, retelling the story of the gun battle that had taken Legend's life. I quickly gathered that Legend had been a prominent drug figure on nearby Chancellor Avenue. I knew the turf well. Homicide detectives who came to investigate were familiar with Legend and they filled me in on his long drug-dealing history. I'm not often surprised, but this news shocked me. Nothing about his wholesome appearance had said drug dealer—no flashy jewelry, no gun, no rolls of money were found when we cut off his clothes. And Legend's dying words were a profession of love for his wife and children. For days, his death was the talk of the hospital. Several of the orderlies, EKG technicians, and nurses knew him or his mother well, and they helped me piece together the legend surrounding Legend.

———

Like so many black boys growing up in Newark, Legend dreamed of making it out, and he knew his ticket would be sports. He was one of those dudes who could do just about all things sports, but he was particularly good at basketball and football. His talents had earned him all-city honors in both sports a couple of times. He received a scholarship to play Division III football at a well-respected university, but to everyone's surprise, he lasted just one semester before returning to the old neighborhood. There he built the drug-dealing empire that ultimately would consume his life. He had ruled the neighborhood without challenge until his mysterious disappearance about a year earlier, when he was a suspect in a high-stakes murder that had occurred in Newark a week before his sudden departure. Police didn't have enough evidence to make a case against Legend and his crew. The no-snitch policy is real in the hood, and often a matter of life and death. You grow up hearing "snitches get stitches," you see evidence of it all the time, and you keep your mouth shut. It's not ideal and not the least bit courageous, but for folks who'd learned the hard way that those hired "to protect and serve" were no match for the thugs on the streets, it's just a matter of survival. The case went unsolved.

"Out of sight, out of mind" is how a relative of Legend's, who was also one of his lieutenants, explained the reason Legend left town. While Legend passed the time at a family member's house in the deep South, there was a rush to claim his highly profitable drug arena, prompting a chain of shootings and stabbings. As I listened to this account of the drug war, I pinpointed the time period instantly. It had been the previous fall, when gunshot victims began showing up in the emergency room every day—so often that we'd felt it necessary to heighten our security.

Legend returned to Newark in early spring 2001 to reclaim his turf. He'd been warned that a new generation, "the young'uns," had taken over, and that they'd earned their ruthless reputation. In their minds, his reign was a thing of the past. Legend was unfazed by his young rivals. He figured he could battle them *and* chop down the former friends who'd become swollen with power in his absence. But the old gangster wasn't coming back to the same streets he'd left. His generation had grown up with a street code that allowed them to return from jail or trips away and reclaim their old spots without much trouble. Others who'd filled the space understood that it was just temporary, and out of respect backed away.

Not so with the young'uns. It was every man for himself. They weren't giving up anything without a battle. They were quick to pull the trigger, and they terrorized Chancellor Avenue with their shooting sprees, killing folks for sport. So they resisted when Legend began to occupy one of the corners with his cadre of runners, lieutenants, deliverers, and lookouts. At first, his return seemed uneventful. He'd gone to school with many of his workers and customers, and he'd spent time in practically every apartment in the neighborhood. Even the police didn't pose much of a threat; Legend knew the officers and their patrol patterns. Some of his young rivals also showed him deference; they'd been groomed by him, after all. They'd grown up running errands for him, back in the day, fetching snacks from the store or chicken dinners from the neighborhood restaurant. In return, they got a few dollars, snacks, chicken dinners for themselves, and, most of all, bragging rights at school the next day.

Before long, Legend had carved out a small niche for himself in his old drug empire and figured the young'uns had just backed away. But on the hot, breezeless day when I met him, the young'uns showed him he'd figured wrong. As the streets tell it, two people on a black motorcycle came rolling down the block where Legend stood talking to his runners. Faceless in black helmets, they pulled up to the corner and opened fire, striking Legend all over his body.

The shooter on the back of the bike then hopped off, walked up to Legend, and taunted: "Where's your lookouts? Know who you got working for you." He then hopped back on the bike and they sped off, leaving a trail of blood on the ground and the smell of burnt rubber in the air.

God only knows how he managed to pull himself up from the sidewalk that should have been his deathbed and stumble to the hospital. For weeks after our lives collided in the E.R., I felt haunted by his confused gaze. His pleading eyes seemed to ask: *How come my cards got played this way?*

It wasn't unusual that I stayed up nights wondering what I could have done differently. Every time I lost a patient, I lost sleep, scrutinizing the lifesaving steps my team had taken, asking myself whether I could have done something better. But Legend's death tore me up like no other. When I saw him in my dreams, it was as though I was looking at myself. I'd wake up sweating . . . and realize that somehow I'd tricked the gods. I'd managed to escape it all—the drugs, the dangerous pursuit of street fame and wealth, early death.

I thought back to a trip I'd taken to the Bronx when I was seventeen, just before the robbery and my time in juvenile detention. My friend Duke—the same Duke who'd masterminded the robbery—had convinced me I could do better than what I was earning working two part-time jobs—one at McDonald's and another at IKEA. Even with both, I never seemed to have enough money to buy the things I needed; of course, I didn't understand then how warped a seventeen-year-old's definition of "need" could be. I'd managed to buy a used Audi 5000, which got me to and from work, but it needed repairs. I didn't have the money, and in the irrational mind of a teenager, fixing my car was a need worth whatever risks I had to take to fulfill it. Duke's nonsense was starting to make sense. We could pool our money and take over the Dayton Street drug trade in no time, he said. If we didn't, someone else would. And so, a short time later, there I was, being patted down inside an Uptown apartment by dudes with Uzis strapped across their chests. Stacks of money and bags of cocaine covered a coffee table. The scene looked like one from a gangster movie, but it was real. So, too, were the risks I hadn't considered before doing this, and the possible consequences. I wanted to turn and walk away, but given the Uzi-toting brothers at the door, I didn't think that would be wise. Duke and I bought the drugs and made a quick exit. A light rain was falling outside, but the droplets felt like slaps across my face. I thought: *What the hell am I doing here?*

The drive back to Newark was nerve-racking. Every time a police car got near us, my heart rate spiked, and I had to remind myself not to speed or draw attention to myself. *How do dudes live like this?* I wondered. It definitely wasn't what I wanted for my life. When we reached home, I told Duke he could have it all. I had no interest in taking over Dayton Street or anywhere else. Drug dealing just wasn't my thing. It would take the robbery and the trip to juvenile detention for me to make a clean break with the thug life, though. Duke, unfortunately, stayed out there, and landed in and out of jail as I struggled through college and medical school.

By the end of my second year of residency at Beth, I was weary of all the bloodshed, weary of pronouncing one young black man after another dead of gunshot wounds, weary of losing to the streets. So when one day in 2001 I encountered yet another young gunshot victim, I'd had enough. He was unconscious, breathing through a tube that had been inserted by emergency medical technicians on the way to the hospital. I cut off his bloody clothes and was peeling away the remnants of his shirt when I noticed a twelve-inch scar. The sight stunned me. It was unmistakably a laparotomy scar, snaking from the pit of his chest to just below his belly button. He had been cut open before. The surgeon standing next to me, Dr. Baker, noticed the scar, too.

"Holy cow!" he exclaimed, moving in to examine it closer. "That's my work."

Baker seemed as certain as if he'd just discovered a long-lost Picasso.

"You took care of this guy before?" I asked, feeling an odd emotion rising inside me.

"Yep, last summer—that's my scar," my colleague replied.

Suddenly, I was ashamed. Most times, I felt empathy for the young brothers, hanging on to life by the thinnest hair after a score had been settled on the streets. I never excused their reckless behavior, but I understood it. Not this time, though. This dude had been shot the previous summer and had experienced a lifesaving operation. Now he was back, in the same position. Dr. Baker, who is white, didn't say another word, but in his silence I heard the judgment of white people (and "bourgie" black folks) everywhere:

"What's wrong with those people?"

Many times I'd found myself explaining to white folks that poverty and crime are not a factor of skin color and that there is nothing about being black or brown that makes a person inherently violent. I'd argued that desperation and hopelessness often make poor people careless about their actions and the consequences. Change the conditions, I'd said, and their lives would change. But as I stood there patching up that guy, my patience and understanding were gone. I wanted to shake him, knock some sense into him, make him really hear me.

What will it take for you to get it, man? I thought. *We don't have to live like this.*

Often in the early years of my residency I wondered: *What had made the difference between me and the many friends I'd lost to drugs and gang violence?* I'd known the same craving that Snake, Duke, and even the repeat offender must have felt for material wealth and respect. I'd known the kind of poverty that often makes a man in that situation feel justified in his wrongdoing—*a man's gotta do what a man's gotta do, take care of himself and take the load off Moms, by any means necessary.* And I'd known the impatience many young brothers feel in a wealth-driven society that they believe is designed for them to fail. In their minds, it's useless to even try playing by the rules. And so they create their own definition of how to win and earn respect.

Consider these disturbing facts: Homicide is the leading cause of death for black men ages fifteen to thirty-four, and most of those murders are committed with firearms, particularly handguns. According to a Bureau of Justice analysis of homicide trends in the United States from 1976 to 2005, African Americans—who made up just 12 to 13 percent of the population during that time—were disproportionately represented among both homicide victims and killers. Nearly 47 percent of all people murdered in the United States in those years were black, as were 52 percent of the killers. And 94 percent of the black victims were killed by other black people.

Even as the homicide rate stabilized nationwide between 1999 and 2005, the number of African American men ages twenty-five to forty-four who were killed by firearms in large cities and suburbs increased a third. And there's more:

- African Americans have the highest rates of deaths by firearms (including homicides, suicides, and unintentional shooting deaths) of all racial groups.
- African American children and teens are five times as likely as their white peers to be killed by firearms.
- African American males, ages fifteen to nineteen, are almost

five times as likely to be killed by firearms as their white peers, and more than twice as likely as their Hispanic and Native American peers.

This long-standing crisis is beyond what law enforcement can handle alone. Children growing up in poor urban neighborhoods aren't programmed by their DNA to run around with guns, killing one another. Violence is learned behavior. And I know from my own experience that the negative lessons learned in an environment saturated by drugs and violence can be unlearned. I also know that so many of our kids who are caught up in this cycle want better. Somehow, we must help them find it.

What Parents Can Do to Help Their Children Avoid Gangs*

- Be close to your children, express affection, and share your values and high expectations for their success in school and life.
- Discuss, clearly and honestly, tough issues, such as alcohol and illegal drugs, smoking, gangs, and sexual involvement.
- Set and enforce reasonable standards of behavior, and praise good behavior.
- Model positive behavior.
- Monitor after-school time and locate after-school programs and mentors for your children.
- Know who your children's friends are and discourage any involvement with gang members, gang clothing, or gang symbols.
- Seek professional help if you suspect your child may be involved with, or threatened by, a gang.

Discussion Questions Parents Might Use with Teens*

- Do they know or have they heard about anyone who has been shot? What happened?
- Do they know about kids at school having guns or being involved in violent activities? What are these kids like? What happened?
- What are their own fears and opinions about guns?
- Have they ever been approached by anyone to buy a gun? How did they respond? How did they feel?
- Have they ever seen a real gun? How did that feel and under what circumstances did this occur?
- Do they feel any pressure to get involved with gun activity?

*Source: Violence Prevention Institute, Inc., 66 West Gilbert Street, Suite 100, Red Bank, NJ 07701

2

HIDDEN IN PLAIN SIGHT

W hen I arrived at Beth Israel in the summer of 1999, eager to do something about the suffering all around me, I was already long familiar with the ways of crack addicts and street junkies. I'd marveled at their lies and their never-ending hustles. I'd seen their love for family, friends, and even God take a backseat to a new god, that white rock or powder, even if all the while they hated themselves for it. Little about that world surprised me anymore. But I was soon introduced to another world, a hidden drug culture right under my nose.

That summer, my first sickle-cell anemia patient showed up in the emergency department during one of my shifts at Beth. He was twenty-three, complaining of pain in his shoulders and upper back. I got excited—in the macabre kind of way that happens when a doctor is about to learn firsthand about an illness or injury he has seen only in textbooks.

Sickle-cell anemia is an inherited blood disorder that in the United States primarily affects African Americans. In a normal patient, red blood cells are oval-shaped, which is optimal for carrying oxygen and allowing blood to flow easily through arteries and veins to the organs and limbs. But a sickle-cell patient has abnormally shaped cells that look like a crescent or sickle. The deformed cells sometimes clump together, blocking the regular flow of blood and oxygen and causing excruciating pain in the deprived areas.

During medical school I studied the disease intensively, since I already knew I wanted to work in an urban hospital, and I figured the illness would show itself time and time again. So on that summer day, I knew all about the illness, but I'd never met anyone with it.

My patient looked like a skinnier version of the actor Wesley Snipes, with dark brown skin, a high-top fade cut close on the sides and back, baggy jeans, and a pair of tan boots. He was writhing on the stretcher.

"Doc, I'm in so much pain," he cried. "I feel like I'm about to die!"

He asked for ten milligrams of Dilaudid, a semi-synthetic version of morphine that is far more potent. Ten milligrams of Dilaudid would have the same effect as about seventy-two milligrams of morphine. That much of such a powerful drug could kill the uninitiated, but to a person in chronic pain who has built up a tolerance for it, the high dosage just brings quick relief. I didn't doubt for a moment that my patient needed it. At his age, he surely had experienced more than a few episodes of sickle-cell pain, which explained in my mind his certainty about the medication and dosage he needed. A quick glance at his chart showed that he'd been given ten milligrams of Dilaudid during his last E.R. visit.

I jumped into rescue mode, assuring the brother that I would take care of him and get him started on the Dilaudid, as well as an oxygen treatment, intravenous fluids, and the Benadryl he'd requested to soothe the itching often caused by histamines released with the medication. I rushed down the hall, found the attending physician, and immediately started describing my patient.

"I have a twenty-three-year-old sickle-cell anemia patient presenting with pain in his shoulder and upper back," I said, full of urgency and earnestness. I mentioned the treatment I wanted to prescribe, in the hope that the attending would sign off quickly. The head doctor's cavalier attitude caught me off guard.

"Oh, that's Thomas Green," he said, chuckling.

His face wore an inexplicable smirk.

"My young doctor," he added, patting me on the back, "you have so much to learn."

I was puzzled. Had I missed something in the diagnosis? The head doctor assured me that this was the right course of treatment for a patient whose pain hadn't responded to lower dosages of the medication or weaker drugs. He approved my recommendation and walked away. Still, his initial response nagged at me. What had his smirk been about? I checked Thomas's chart again, this time more carefully. Sure enough, he'd been given ten milligrams of Dilaudid during his last emergency room visit—as a matter of fact, during his last several visits. I slowed down, looking closely at their dates, and my jaw dropped. Thomas had shown up at the hospital in crisis at least fifteen times in the past month. Even for a sickle-cell anemia patient, that was excessive. No wonder the attending physician knew immediately who he was. And no wonder my supervisor found my sincerity laughable. This dude seemed to be running a game.

But how could I be sure?

Therein lies the doctor's dilemma. We can diagnose illness, and we can identify the conditions that generally cause pain. But we cannot quantify pain. Medical professionals have long defined it in the same way registered nurse and pain management expert Margo McCaffery described it in 1968: Pain is "whatever the experiencing person says it is, existing whenever and wherever the person says it does."

So now, despite my suspicions, I could not say with 100 percent certainty that Thomas was faking in order to get the drugs. I could have costly tests run to show there were no other ailments, but that wouldn't prove there was no pain. Sometimes, even when we've done every test known to science, and they show no reason for pain to exist, it still does. Much of medicine remains mysterious; new discoveries are made every day. As a physician, I never want to see anyone suffer. My fulfillment comes in healing and easing pain and suffering. The last thing I want to do is make an unfounded accusation against someone who is genuinely suffering. There was another issue that concerned me, too: race and stereotyping. Thomas was African American, and I didn't want to assume that he was lying to get a fix. As an African American man, I know what it's like to walk into a room and feel the vibes of people who are making assumptions before they know the first thing about you.

I stood there reading his chart and reasoning. Thomas had a genuine disease, a painful disease, and I saw he had suffered mightily. Diminished blood flow to his hip tissues and bone had caused a degenerative condition called "avascular necrosis," which had required him to undergo hip replacement surgery. His spleen had been removed after a buildup of sickled cells had caused a splenic sequestration—an enlarged spleen. And Thomas certainly appeared to be in pain now as he lay curled up on the stretcher. His chart indicated not only his tolerance for the drug but the decision many doctors before me had made to give it to him. So I followed suit and administered the Dilaudid.

About two hours later, making my way through the unit where Thomas had been assigned, I saw him sleeping soundly. Walking down the hallway, I accidentally bumped into his stretcher, which was pushed against a wall. He jolted straight up, looked at the clock, and said, "Hey, Doc, glad you're here. I need more pain medicine."

Beth Israel had a rule: Dilaudid and other narcotics of that type could be administered no more than once every two hours, and ten milligrams was the maximum dose that doctors were allowed to prescribe in the E.R. Thomas had awakened from a sound sleep already needing more pain medicine? He'd timed his request almost to the minute. With a string of emergencies vying for my time, I couldn't stand there debating whether this guy was in real pain or playing me for a fool. "I'll send a nurse to help you," I said, dashing off to the next patient. Thomas would request a third dose, the maximum allowed without being admitted, before suddenly feeling well enough to go home. The attending physician's words echoed in my head: *My young doctor, you have so much to learn.*

So began my education into the underworld of the E.R. Thomas showed up at the emergency department at least twice a week, same routine. What little faith I had in his sincerity began to fade, especially as I noticed the same suspicious behavior among about a half-dozen other patients, whom I came to know as the "sickle-cell posse."

Ann and LaShawn were friends in their mid-twenties who probably had met in Beth Israel's emergency department. When one would show up, claiming to be experiencing the worst pain of her life, the staff came to expect that within a half hour, the other would make her way there as well. Ann, short and slim, would stroll in, usually dressed in jeans, a T-shirt, and sneakers. She had a long, reddish-colored weave flowing down her back. And less than thirty minutes later, on cue, there was LaShawn, also short and thin, with gold streaks in dark hair that she kept mostly hidden under a baseball cap. They always asked to be assigned beds next to each other, and they'd bring nail polish and other beauty products to share. Since they were there for six hours or more at a time, they'd traipse up and down the hall to the vending machines, buying chips and sodas. As I passed them, I'd see the two sitting on one bed, their supplies spread out between them, giving each other manicures and pedicures, or braiding each other's hair, like they were on summer vacation. Or they'd just sit there, chatting, dangling their legs, talking on their cell phones, and watching the clock.

Precisely two hours after getting their first meds, they'd raise their hands, like they were in school. "Doc, I'm due for my second round of pain medicine," one of them would state, as if the next dose was supposed to be automatic. And after their third dose, they would say they were better and ready to go home. Hospital rules required me to admit a patient who showed no progress after the third dose. None of the so-called "frequent fliers" wanted to be admitted. Overnight stays in the hospital meant more regular monitoring and lower dosages of the narcotics over longer periods, and it completely cramped their itinerant style.

The gall of their assumptions angered me. I thought, *You're not automatically due for a second round of drugs; you're allowed a second round* if you're in pain. *And how much pain can you be in right now, painting toenails?*

One day, a nurse who doubled at other hospitals was working her shift at Beth Israel when she recognized the pair of friends and exclaimed, "Oh my God, that's Ann and LaShawn—I just saw them yesterday at University Hospital!"

It came as no surprise to anyone that the two women E.R.-shopped, visiting emergency rooms throughout the area to get drugs. An addict will go wherever and whenever to get her next fix. The drugs are also quite valuable on the street, and so a prescription could be a moneymaker.

The hospital tried mightily to help patients with chronic pain, and, of course, those who abused narcotics represented just a small portion of the ones treated for pain in the emergency department. And let me be clear: Not all sickle-cell patients are drug seekers. Likewise, not all drug seekers are sickle-cell patients. During practically every shift at least one patient came into the E.R. complaining of severe back pain, a toothache, a migraine, or some mysterious pain and offering a story that raised suspicions: His regular doctor was out of town, or her medicine was misplaced, or he was vacationing in the area and had left his medication at home. They usually asked for the narcotics by name: Dilaudid, morphine, OxyContin, Percocet were among the more popular ones.

Sometimes they even put on Oscar-worthy performances, like the guy who was brought by ambulance one day from the Newark train station. He was supposedly traveling back home to Massa-. chusetts from Texas, and while on a layover in Newark he experienced what witnesses described as a seizure. He reported to our staff a past history of chronic back pain but no prior seizures. While being observed and awaiting the results of blood work, the patient again began convulsing. The resident on duty moved fast to administer medication, likely Ativan, to control the seizure. I rushed to the patient's bedside. For several minutes, his body shook. But one thing stood out: He never let go of the bed's handrail. Normally, a person having a grand mal seizure loses total body control and is incapable of holding or grasping anything. I opened his eyelids, and his eyes followed me. I knew exactly what was going on. I leaned over and whispered in his ear, "Stop it, I know you're faking." He didn't respond.

It was rarely that easy to determine when a patient was just seeking drugs, though. Among the "frequent fliers," having a documentable disease made the hustle easier. And it soon became clear to me that prescription drug abuse, once the nasty little secret of the rich and famous, was now a huge twenty-first-century problem in urban neighborhoods. These new addicts weren't hiding out in abandoned houses, shooting up behind closed doors; their drugs of choice were administered by professionals in the cool, clean corridors of the E.R. And the unwitting dealers in this game weren't working the streets with Glocks hidden in their pants, they had fancy degrees and wore white lab coats. That's what bothered me the most: I started to feel like a high-class drug dealer.

When I mentioned to Ann and LaShawn that they'd been spotted in the emergency room at University Hospital the previous day, neither seemed fazed. Both said something like, "I was in pain, and University was close to where I was."

So I treated them. I felt I had no choice. Number one, I didn't want to take the risk of failing to treat a patient who was really in pain. State law requires that I provide medical care to everyone who comes to the hospital seeking it, and I couldn't prove that these patients were *not* in pain. The hospital staff lived with the constant fear that a patient would complain to the state about being denied treatment, which could trigger an investigation and result in the hospital getting cited and potentially facing cuts to its Medicare/Medicaid funding. With dwindling resources forcing hospitals throughout the country to close their emergency rooms or shut down altogether, the threat felt very real. It was easier just to write the prescription.

Our pharmacy network lent a hand in helping to keep track of how many times a particular medication had been prescribed to an individual patient. Repeated narcotic prescriptions always raise a red flag, particularly if they come from different doctors. I received calls on numerous occasions from pharmacists alerting me that someone who had left the emergency department with a prescription written by me had recently been prescribed sixty tablets of the same medication by a doctor at another medical facility.

Then the pharmacist would ask: "Dr. Davis, do you still want me to fill the script?"

My response was always the same: "No, and I will notify my department so they're on the lookout."

There were times I tried to claim small moral victories, quietly reducing the dosage of the pain medication the staff administered to a patient I suspected of abuse, or refusing to send the patient home with a prescription for Percocet or OxyContin. Other times, I refused to give the third dose of Dilaudid, insisting instead that if the patient was still in pain, he needed to be admitted into the hospital. My refusal to follow the unwritten rules occasionally resulted in blowups. A patient would protest loudly, curse me out, and sometimes even trail me around the department, threatening to call the state to complain about poor treatment and a lack of respect.

That was sort of how I wound up one sunny spring day in 2002 sitting in the emergency medical director's office. The discussion was to be my quarterly Patient Satisfaction Review, a survey that had become the latest trend in hospitals' frantic quest to generate business in an era of budget cuts and reduced services. How satisfied a hospital's patients were played a large part in its reputation. My scores, normally above average, had fallen a bit, I suspected because of my growing impatience with drug seekers. I arrived early for the meeting, and Dr. Fink's secretary was kind enough to allow me to wait in his office. With coffee in hand, I stood mesmerized by the degrees, board certificates, and awards filling his wall. The office, located on the top floor of the hospital, offered a panoramic view of the Newark skyline, a sea of tall brick buildings interspersed with small patches of green. Far off in the distance, you could see New York City. Less than a year earlier, I'd watched the aftermath of the September 11 terrorist attacks from this window.

As I waited, I rehearsed in my head what I would say when Dr. Fink instructed me to be less confrontational. I would hear him out without agreeing to change my position. I would point to literature showing the rise in prescription drug abuse. I was not a drug dealer.

I glanced at the framed photos on the director's mahogany desk. There were pictures of his family, his dog, and buddies dressed in army fatigues. I recalled Dr. Fink saying once that he was an army dude. I leaned in a bit to look more closely at a photo of him with his two sons, a black-and-white shot that had been taken outside, maybe while fishing or camping. The boys appeared to be close in age and tall and slim, like their father. Suddenly, without warning, Dr. Fink, a man in his fifties with just the right amount of salt-and-pepper hair to equal his experience, entered his office. Embarrassed, I straightened from my detective position over his desk.

Moving to his chair, he sat and motioned for me to take a seat across from him, which I did. He then said: "How are things, Sampson?"

"Things are well, Dr. Fink. No complaints," I responded, keeping my cool.

"You know, Sampson, medicine is a great field," he began, then continued for a few moments, talking about how doctors gain extraordinary wisdom from what we see in the field.

I nodded in agreement, waiting to hear where he was going with this conversation. We both were busy. And he hadn't called the meeting to talk about the joys of medicine. Dr. Fink must've seen in my eyes that I was eager to get on with it, because he quickly got to the point. "Sampson, do you know why you're here?"

Again, I nodded.

"Well, let's just say, when you're dealing with cases that are not actual emergencies, try to imagine one that truly moved you. I know you have plenty, so I won't ask you."

He paused. I was puzzled, and feeling a bit like I was in the principal's office—I half expected my mother to come tearing through the door any minute, belt in hand.

I asked, "Is that it?"

"Yes, that's it. Take care."

Still slightly confused, I rose from my seat and left the office. Dr. Fink was a child of the seventies. Had I just experienced a hippie moment? *Live peacefully and think of memorable cases.* I laughed quietly all the way back down to the emergency department. It was an unexpectedly light moment in a frustrating scenario.

I often referred—or tried to refer—patients to the hospital's social worker for pain-management counseling or to the psychiatry department for narcotics-abuse treatment, with the hope that they would get the help they truly needed. But there was not enough staff to handle the need, and there were rarely any available beds in the psych ward. And even when a room opened up, the patient held the upper hand: Nothing was mandatory. If he denied having a drug problem, he could refuse an intervention or check himself out of the hospital at any time, which is what usually happened. Beth Israel's pain-management counseling tried to address the issue broadly, but many patients wouldn't show up for scheduled sessions or refused to even make an appointment. Many patients didn't see themselves as addicts. In their minds, an addict was the crackhead uncle begging for money on the corner or the strung-out sister pawning their parents' possessions.

Because of the staff's heightened suspicions, I'm sure there were times when patients who were hurting and needed relief were wrongly viewed as addicts, as well as times when addicts with real illnesses were indeed in pain. In those cases, they most likely received the appropriate medication and treatment, but perhaps with a little less compassion than they deserved. That is one of the heartbreaking fallouts of this dilemma.

No one was suspicious of Mr. Jacobs, though. He was an Afrocentric, Malcolm X–looking dude in his late fifties who usually wore an African dashiki and matching kufi cap. A couple of times I saw him receiving treatment in the emergency room late at night in his pajamas and robe. He carried himself in a dignified manner, and the staff treated him with deference and respect.

When I first met Mr. Jacobs in 2002, he mentioned the memoir I'd just written with George and Rameck. "Man, I heard about you young brothers," he told me. "You're doing great things in the community."

At his age, Mr. Jacobs seemed like a modern miracle. He had lived more than a decade past the life expectancy of a man with sickle-cell anemia. (The average for a man with the disease is forty-two years; for a woman, forty-eight.) Mr. Jacobs kept up with the latest news, and whenever I saw him at the hospital, he talked about the racial politics of the disease, the need for more research, and how sickle-cell anemia always seemed to draw the short end of the stick when it came to government funding. The latest statistics and research rolled off his tongue. Mr. Jacobs told me that he had founded a small support group for sickle-cell anemia patients and their families and asked if I would speak at a future meeting. I agreed without hesitation. But we never nailed down a specific day. One thing seemed a little odd to me: For someone who had founded a group on behalf of those stricken with the disease, Mr. Jacobs never seemed to mingle with any of the other sickle-cell patients. *Maybe he's suspicious of some of them because they seek drug treatment so frequently,* I thought. *Maybe he's worried that their actions might reflect badly on his group.*

Sometime later, Mr. Jacobs was admitted to the hospital. The internist on duty that day ran a series of blood tests, including a routine screening for sickle-cell anemia. When the results came back, everyone was shocked: Mr. Jacobs did not have the disease; instead, he was simply a carrier of the trait, which in most cases causes no symptoms, or minor ones, such as anemia. Over the past decade, researchers have found that in rare cases, a person with the trait may experience severe exhaustion, greater rates of urinary tract and kidney infections, and, in isolated instances, even episodes of pain similar to the disease. Was Mr. Jacobs an anomaly? Or was he just a more dignified drug addict? I will never be certain, and as far as I know, nothing ever changed with his treatment. That's the most maddening part of the dilemma.

There have been hopeful moments, though, like when I met fifteen-year-old Patrick. He was the color of cedar, with bright, happy eyes—and he was also the size of an average ten-year-old. The lack of adequate blood flow throughout the body sometimes stunts the growth of sickle-cell patients. Patrick's mother, Janice, brought him to the emergency room one day with debilitating pain in his back and knees. He could barely walk.

Janice was in her mid-to-late thirties, with a bubbly, young personality. She seemed hip to the latest styles of clothes—looking put together in her jeans, heels, and leather jacket. More important, I could tell by the thorough way she answered my questions that she was hands-on with both her son and his medical care. She explained that she'd given him ibuprofen and his prescribed pills earlier, when he'd first complained of pain, but he hadn't gotten any better. After examining Patrick, I told them I'd decided to start him on a small dose of morphine. His mother interrupted.

"Oh, no, Dr. Davis!" she said. "Don't give him morphine." She asked if he could start his treatment with Toradol, a non-narcotic anti-inflammatory prescription pain reliever similar to ibuprofen. But Toradol comes in a liquid that can be administered through an

IV, which some patients believe brings relief faster than a pill. "He usually does fine with it," she added.

While Patrick's pain certainly seemed severe enough to merit the morphine, his mother had the insight to know that giving him narcotics too soon could be problematic later. I wanted to hug her. With her involvement, he had a better-than-average chance of staying on track.

Patrick reminded me of another teenager, Wayne, whom I'd met in 1999, my first year of residency, when I worked on the pediatric side of the department.

The basic facts matched. Wayne, too, was an African American teenager with sickle-cell anemia, and had come to the hospital with a woman, who I presumed was his mother. But that's where the similarity ends. As I examined Wayne, the woman seemed to fade into the background. And when I asked about his pain or prior medications, he responded himself.

A short, round dude, he was unusually thick for a sickle-cell patient. His hair was braided in neat little cornrows; after that first visit, it was braided in a different style nearly every time I saw him. That day, Wayne was experiencing serious pain in his back and knees. I treated him with a dose of Toradol until the pain subsided. The teenager was upbeat and chatty, even in pain. The few times a year I saw him after that, I'd treat him with the maximum amount of Toradol and release him when the pain subsided. If his pain didn't respond to the Toradol, I added a small bit of morphine. That approach seemed to work well; it kept the narcotics to a minimum and eased his pain. This is a common strategy in treating young patients with chronic pain.

When Wayne turned eighteen, I could no longer treat him on the pediatrics side. He was moved into the department's general population, and he came to the hospital alone. It was not uncommon to have three or four sickle-cell anemia patients receiving treatment at the same time on any given day; whenever possible, the medical staff grouped them together to make the frequent monitoring more convenient for the nurses. Because of crowding and the reality that sickle-cell patients were usually there all day, their stretchers most often were lined up, head to foot, against the wall on the O side of the hallway, the observation area for stable patients. I began to notice Wayne mingling with the others.

It didn't take long before he started showing up in the emergency room more frequently—changing from every few months to once a month to every other week. Then he began complaining that the Toradol wasn't easing his pain at all. I wasn't on duty each time he came to the emergency room, so I didn't see it personally, but his chart told the story: one milligram of Dilaudid, then two, then four, and on and on. In just over a year, Wayne had gone from taking almost no narcotics to receiving ten milligrams of Dilaudid, the maximum dose. And the newest member of the posse learned well. He began instructing the duty doctor on how much medication he needed, and if the doctor ordered less, Wayne would follow him or a nurse around the department, demanding: "This is not my proper dose. I am in pain, and you need to give me my proper dose!"

By the time Wayne turned twenty, he had progressed to taking three rounds of the maximum dose of Dilaudid. One day, after his third dose, he said he was still in pain. He agreed to be admitted to the hospital and was transferred to an inpatient room. During one of her rounds, the nurse found Wayne lying motionless in bed. His chest wasn't rising. She felt for his pulse. Nothing. His skin, normally a golden color, now appeared dull and dusky. She buzzed the nurse's station, which called a Code Blue, and within seconds the medical response team was at his side, working to resuscitate him.

But it was too late. Wayne was dead.

It was spring 2002, and when I arrived at work the next day, the staff was still buzzing with the news and speculation on what had happened.

"Did you hear about Wayne?" someone asked, then filled me in.

I was startled. Even though I'd watched from a distance Wayne's tragic transformation from sick kid to drug addict, I hadn't seen this coming. There were rumors that he had either cocaine or heroin in his system as well as the Dilaudid that final day, or that he'd injected a street drug into his IV, trying for a faster, more intense high. As far-fetched as that may seem, there had been a similar incident in 2000, late in my first year on the job.

That patient also had sickle-cell; but, in addition, he bore a laparotomy scar from some type of surgery to his abdomen. The few times I'd encountered him in the emergency department, he was rubbing his belly, complaining of severe pain in his scar area. He was a grumpy dude, who barked orders at the staff: "Gimme my pain medicine, now!" His last day, he was in a room on the inpatient side when the nurse found him, unresponsive. A bottle of Robitussin was at his bedside. The staff suspected he had injected the cough syrup into his IV.

I never learned for sure what happened in either suspicious death. At the time, I was shocked. But recent studies show that prescription drug abuse is the fastest growing drug problem in the United States, and deaths from overdoses of prescription painkillers are on the rise. In a November 2011 report that examined such deaths from 1999 to 2008, the Centers for Disease Control and Prevention called the problem an epidemic, saying that prescription drugs are behind the overall increase in drug overdose deaths. Even more startling, a greater number of people are dying from overdoses of prescription drugs, such as OxyContin and Vicodin, than from cocaine and heroin overdoses combined. The rise in prescription drug overdose deaths has been so steep that by 2008, they were approaching the number of deaths from motor vehicle crashes, the leading cause of injury death in the United States.

A few weeks after Wayne died, I learned that another of our sickle-cell patients was his sister. Her name was Sarah, and she was in her mid-twenties, a few years older than Wayne. She had come to the emergency department for pain treatment that day and mentioned she had been struggling with depression since her brother's death. Though Sarah and Wayne shared the same last name and had similar features—short and round with gold-colored skin—I'd never seen them together and hadn't until that moment made the connection that they were siblings.

"I didn't realize Wayne was your brother," I told her. "I'm really sorry about what happened."

Sarah, who always spoke in a soft, babyish voice, seemed distant and withdrawn. After that day, I noticed, she began careening downhill. I'd sometimes catch a glimpse of her, looking haggard and beaten down, a baseball cap or scarf pulled over her head, in a drug-induced sleep—or sitting in a daze on a hallway stretcher. This was doubly sad. Not only did both siblings have the same terrible, life-shortening disease, they both became addicted to pain-killers . . . and perhaps more. I knew nothing about the siblings' lives and struggles beyond the hospital, but I grappled with this question: Did we do more harm than good? We were supposed to help our patients, or at least do no harm. That's what all doctors promise when we take the Hippocratic Oath.

As time went on, I grew more and more vocal among my colleagues with my complaints about the drug seekers and the anguish I felt prescribing narcotics when I had serious doubts about whether the patient needed it. One day, a fellow doctor blurted: "Just write the prescription. Why do you even care?"

I pondered that question the rest of the day: Why *did* I care?

The answer boiled down to this, I realized: When I was a naïve, impatient teenager, I'd walked away from drug dealing. I'd left behind the deceit and danger associated with that life and held on to hope that there was something better for me. I'd gripped every hand that reached down to pull me up and out. And no way had I come this far to end up in a fancy version of the hell I'd left behind.

At the moment, I wasn't sure what, if anything, I could do. But I knew this: Remaining silent was no longer an option.

3

BRICK CITY

My exhausting twelve-hour shift at Beth was just a minute from ending one day in 2003 when I found myself in the center of a tragic reproductive mystery. The previous night had been a breeze—a few runny noses, a dog bite, and a couple of pediatric ear infections. As I glanced up at the clock one final time, the doors to my left swung open, and my replacement, Dr. Jones, strolled in, looking fresh and ready to take control. All I had left to do was sign out my two remaining patients, one of whom had an upset stomach that I was hydrating with saline and the other a heart patient with chest pains that we were monitoring closely.

In emergency medicine, the sooner you master the overnight shift, the better. But no matter how many times I worked it, I just never got used to staying up all night. This day was no exception. My brain had reached overdrive, and my red, bleary eyes gave away my exhaustion. I was just about to bid my colleagues goodbye when I heard a commotion brewing to my right. Looking past the tight circle of nurses, technicians, and residents, I managed to make out a woman slouched in a wheelchair being rushed into the department. Her head was flung backward, and her arms hung limply at her sides. She looked pregnant and appeared to be un-

conscious. Instincts and adrenaline kicked in. Only a few feet separated me from Dr. Jones, who was moving toward us, but in
matters of life and death, seconds are crucial. I was closer, so I
sped to the patient's side.

She appeared to be in her early-to-mid-thirties and about thirty
to thirty-five weeks pregnant. As the staff lifted her from the
wheelchair onto a stretcher in the resuscitation room, I started my
rapid-fire battery of questions.

"What happened?" I yelled in the frenzy.

My colleagues chimed in what they'd been able to piece together
quickly when they ran to the door after hearing her husband's
frantic pounding on the emergency room window: She'd suddenly
started having trouble breathing at home, and as her husband was
rushing her to the hospital, she lost consciousness. An emergency
room respiratory technician delivered oxygen through a bag valve
mask, a lifesaving device used to push air into the lungs. I instructed the junior resident to take over and the senior resident to
prepare for intubation, the placement of a breathing tube into the
patient's windpipe or trachea. In search of a pulse, I placed my
right hand on her femoral artery, one of the major blood vessels
located in the upper thigh—but I felt nothing. I heard no heartbeat
through my stethoscope either. There was no chest wall movement, no breathing. I started CPR and yelled for a nurse to page
the obstetricians. An E.R. technician pulled a metal footstool to
the side of the stretcher, jumped atop it, and started pushing on the
patient's chest, performing compressions as if his own life de-
pended on it. This would help circulate the blood throughout the
patient's body and deliver it to her vital organs—the heart, brain,
and kidneys—as well as to the unborn child. We had to get her
blood moving; it was our only hope. The wait for the obstetricians
seemed to take forever, but they arrived in only about two minutes, panting from their sprint to the emergency department. They

recognized the medical emergency right away. Seconds later, they were gloved, scalpels in hand.

The only chance of survival for both the child and mother was to deliver the baby immediately via C-section. Normally the surgery is performed with general anesthesia in a sterile operating room, but there was no time. It had to be done right then to allow the child a chance to breathe on its own. The obstetricians made a straight incision from the top of the patient's abdomen down to her belly button. They cut the uterus in a similar fashion, pulled the baby from the womb, and cut the umbilical cord. It was a boy. His dusky purple skin was covered with blood and amniotic fluid. Miraculously, we managed to get a slight pulse and heartbeat, but even after we administered oxygen, the infant's color remained dull. A nurse paged the neonatal doctor, who arrived shortly for a more thorough examination. I watched closely as the infant was placed onto warm sheets in an incubator and rolled away to the Neonatal Intensive Care Unit.

As the obstetricians did their part, tending to the baby, I did mine, caring for the mother. We tried epinephrine and atropine, squeezed a saline fluid through the central line, and kept up the chest compressions. Still, we got no response, no blood pressure, no spontaneous respirations, not even a flicker of life. There wasn't a soul in the room who didn't feel the weight of the situation, and no one was giving up. But unlike on television, the cardiac monitor didn't suddenly start chirping after all the heroic medical measures. This wasn't Hollywood. This was Newark. This was real life, and the flat line on the monitor wasn't flinching. Sweat was now pouring from our foreheads, and all eyes remained fixed on the patient. But as the truth became evident, a few eyes began turning toward the floor. Our patient was dead. She had been dead when she'd arrived. I'd known it then but had been hopeful we could somehow trick death and snatch her back. I pronounced her dead at 7:45 A.M.

Her husband was out in the waiting room, completely unaware. I asked a nurse to escort him to the family room, a more private place for relatives to receive news about their loved ones. The windowless room with its white walls and uninspiring canvas painting felt sterile and cold, but it was at least secluded. I stripped off my bloody gloves, scrubbed my hands, and took a deep breath, preparing for the most dreaded part of my job. The nurse soon returned with news that the husband was in the family room with two small children.

"What?" I blurted. "Two kids?"

As if her death were not tragic enough, she had two other children who had just lost their mother? What could I say to her husband? My head was pounding as I headed for the small room where they were waiting. I stepped inside and noticed two boys, who appeared to be about three and five years old, hugging the father's legs. Both boys had to be the couple's children; they were the spitting image of their mother. My presence made them uncomfortable, and they tried to hide their faces. I made eye contact with their father, Mr. Thomas, who looked up at me with an expression of fear mixed with hope that I'd never seen before. I stuck my right hand out to introduce myself.

Instead, he grabbed my shoulders and demanded, "Is she okay? Please, Doctor, tell me she's all right."

Before I could respond, he continued speaking, quickly, describing what had happened at the family's home before he brought his wife to the hospital: "She said she couldn't breathe, and I called the ambulance, but they never came. We waited and waited, but they never came. She looked like she was getting worse, so I took her to the car and drove her here as fast as I could. Tell me she's all right! Tell me I did the right thing!"

I jumped in to assure him: "You did. You did do the right thing," I said.

His words kept flowing. And the more I learned, the angrier I became that the city's emergency medical system had failed this woman. She was a nurse, and she was in the final two weeks of her pregnancy, her husband said. The family lived in Newark, and he'd dialed 911 several times. Each time, a dispatcher informed him that an ambulance was on the way. Finally, he loaded his wife and children into the car, racing to the closest hospital. On the way, he could see his wife struggling to breathe, and just minutes before they made it to Beth Israel, she went limp. He kept calling her name, but she didn't respond. He pulled up to the ambulance bay, jumped out of the car, and knocked on the window of the emergency department so hard that only the thickness of the glass had kept it from shattering.

Knowing how desperately Mr. Thomas had tried to save his wife only made the news I was about to deliver even more tragic. I'd needed to sit for this conversation, but Mr. Thomas had rushed over to me with the boys in tow.

"We did everything we possibly could," I began, "and you have a new seven-pound baby boy. He was delivered by one of the fastest cesareans I've ever seen. Miraculously, we were able to get a pulse and blood pressure. He's very sick, but he's hanging on."

I paused. "But your wife, she was unresponsive," I said, continuing. "We did everything we could."

The gravity of the situation seemed to wash over him. "What are you saying? My wife is dead?" He shook his head, looked at his sons, then to me again. "Are you sure?"

I nodded slightly. "Yes. Mr. Thomas, I'm very, very sorry."

His expression, or lack thereof, is something I will never forget. An empty stare with depths beyond the ocean floor is the best way I can describe it. He looked at me with the saddest eyes.

"What am I to do?" he asked. "Tell me, what am I to do?"

"Mr. Thomas, you have a newborn son and two other little

boys who need you now more than ever. I know it is difficult, but you have to be strong."

My words meant little. "You can take the baby," he told me. "Without my wife, I can't do it. I need my wife." He looked around the room, and back to me once more, almost frantically. "Give me my wife! What am I supposed to do?"

I had no answers. All I could muster was a meager "one day at a time." Mr. Thomas collapsed onto the striped beige sofa. Everything about his life had just changed with unbelievable abruptness. I knew he needed a moment alone with his children to grieve. I again expressed my sorrow, then left to call the medical examiner. Since Mrs. Thomas was a young woman with no known disease, her body would be held for an autopsy. Tests would have to be performed to determine the cause of death. I had absolutely no idea what they would reveal. Nothing made sense.

When I returned to the family room, Mr. Thomas was curled in a fetal position on the sofa; the children stood next to him. He opened his eyes and begged, "Please give me my wife's body. Let me take her home." He rose slowly and described a ritual that had been performed for generations in his native Haiti to loosen the seriously ill from the grip of death—prayers, a chant with a hymn, water and oils sprinkled over the loved one's body. "I've never tried it, but I know it will work," he pleaded. "Please give her body to me. I have to take her now if there's any hope.

"I cannot take care of my children without my wife," he continued. "I need my wife! How will the new baby survive without his mother?"

His words weighed on me. My shift was over, and so I just sat with him. I explained that the medical rules would not allow me to let him take his wife's body home but that he would be allowed to see her and say good-bye. He was clearly on the edge emotionally, but I managed to get names and contact information for additional family members. The staff kept their eyes on his children. The boys had just lost their mother and now watched in confusion as their father fell apart. Soon, other grief-stricken family members began to arrive. They were understandably in shock and repeatedly asked the same question that was on my mind: How did this happen? When I finally left the hospital, Mr. Thomas had been admitted for an overnight stay and was being sedated.

Later that night I returned to the hospital for my next shift and received a tragic update: The baby had died, too. The poor child had never stood a chance. He'd spent his short time alive experiencing multiple complications, including seizures and periods of unresponsiveness. Those few minutes without oxygen had caused irreversible damage to his organs. I wanted to attend Mrs. Thomas's funeral. Even though she most likely had died before she'd reached the emergency room, I felt connected to her.

She was a fellow medical professional who had chosen to live in the city over the suburbs, a rare choice among young professionals working in Newark at the time. In the decades after the 1967 riots, census records show, Newark had lost 100,000 residents, mostly middle-income, both white and black. It was a devastating drain of talent and resources. By the time I returned home in 1999, though, the city seemed to be inching back toward a long-promised revitalization.

Politicians had finally figured out that packing poor families on top of one another in huge, poorly maintained high-rise complexes only increased crime. So the 1960s-style public housing projects that had helped to give Newark the moniker "Brick City" were being imploded and replaced by garden townhouses. But what would this revitalization mean if the city couldn't provide basic services to protect residents like Mrs. Thomas, who'd decided that life in the city was worth the trouble?

Unfortunately, the medical examiner's report shed no new light on her death. It said only that she'd died of cardiac arrest. I already knew that; I was the one who'd written it on her chart. What I wanted to know was why: *Why* had her heart stopped? Why had a previously healthy young mother suddenly stopped breathing? I researched the possibilities and suspected a blood clot, or what's called an "amniotic fluid embolism," a rare condition in which amniotic fluid or fetal hair, cells, or other debris somehow get caught up in the circulation of the mother's blood flow from her heart to her lungs, causing both organs to shut down abruptly.

There's no telling how many minutes really had passed from the time Mr. Thomas first called 911 to the moment he decided they could no longer wait for help. In a crisis, passing seconds can seem like an eternity. And when a patient goes into cardiac arrest, every moment is crucial. The time it takes for help to arrive can mean the difference between life and death. A patient can die, or suffer permanent brain damage, if not treated within four to six minutes of the heart stopping.

And too often, emergency help doesn't arrive quickly enough. An investigation published in 2005 by *USA Today* found that emergency medical systems in fifty of the country's largest cities are slow and inconsistent and save only a small fraction of the victims who would be saved with the help of improved response times. A myriad of problems—infighting and turf wars between fire departments and ambulance services, inconsistent ways of measuring performance and response times, the lack of leadership around the issue—contribute to the delays, the investigation found. Cities that have addressed these issues head-on and improved the true time from the initial call for help to the delivery of medical services save many more lives.

I will never know for sure whether any of these potential problems contributed to Mrs. Thomas's death. But I am haunted by the thought that a young mother who spent her days helping to save lives had no one there to save hers in the moments that mattered most. In the end, I decided against attending her funeral. I worried that my presence might only pile on to the family's grief, reminding them of that fateful day in the emergency room when their lives changed suddenly and forever.

I never expected to learn what happened next in the family's life. But about a year later, I was working an emergency room shift at another hospital when I entered the room of a patient who had sprained his shoulder lifting a heavy object. As soon as I walked in, I recognized the man accompanying my patient. It was clear from his expression that he recognized me, too. It was Mr. Thomas. I had never forgotten his face, or his raw grief. All of a sudden, we were back to that awful night. I wasn't sure what he would say. But his face softened into a smile, and before I could utter a word, he spoke.

"Thank you, Doctor," he said, extending his hand. "Thank you for all you did."

I asked about the children. They were well, he said. He looked well, too. I smiled and gripped his hand tightly, greatly relieved, and grateful for this rare moment of closure.

Symptoms of Sudden Cardiac Arrest

- Chest pains
- Weakness
- Shortness of breath or inability to breathe normally
- Heart palpitations
- Vomiting
- Sudden collapse or unresponsiveness
- Loss of consciousness
- No pulse

What to Do If You Encounter Someone Who Has Collapsed or Is Unresponsive

- Call 911 (or your area's emergency response system)
- Conduct CPR. If the person isn't breathing, press hard and fast on his/her chest (a hundred compressions per minute). If you've been trained in CPR, deliver rescue breaths after every thirty compressions. If you haven't, continue chest compressions, allowing the chest to rise completely between each. Keep doing this until emergency help arrives or a portable defibrillator becomes available.
- Use a portable defibrillator (if available). If you have not been trained how to use it, inform the 911 or emergency operator, who may be able to walk you through the process. Deliver one shock (if advised by the device) and begin CPR with chest compressions for about two minutes. Using the defibrillator, check the person's heart rhythm. If necessary, the defibrillator will administer a shock. Repeat until the patient regains consciousness or EMS personnel arrive.

4

LOVE HURTS

I always took a moment to steel myself whenever I picked up a chart outside a room on the A side of the department. This was the obstetrics and gynecology side, though crowding sometimes landed a woman there because we had nowhere else to put her. I learned quickly that behind those doors, marked A1 to A4, tending to a woman's pain often required a different sensitivity than, say, fixing a broken arm.

I'd been on the job less than a year that day in early spring 2000 when I walked into A4 and saw the woman I came to know as Debra sitting there. Something about her made me instantly suspicious. It wasn't just her bruised and swollen face, which looked as if she had been punched. And it wasn't the deep gash on her forehead, which left a bloody trail to her scalp and matted a patch of her shoulder-length black hair to her head. Those injuries could have happened the way she'd described to the triage nurse: in a clumsy tumble into her bedroom dresser. But her uneasiness, the way she seemed to want to disappear when I walked into the examining room, told me there was more to her story.

Sitting upright on the examining table with her feet dangling over the side, she stared at the floor, carefully avoiding my eyes. She tugged at the paper gown, pulling it around her chest to hide as much skin as possible. I wondered why she seemed so nervous, like a child harboring a secret that was about to be exposed. When I asked what had happened, she repeated the same story she'd told the triage nurse: She'd fallen and hit her head on her bedroom dresser. But as she stretched out so I could take a closer look at her injuries, I noticed fresh bruises on her arms and legs—injuries that didn't seem consistent with the fall she'd just described.

I placed my stethoscope on her chest and heard her heart thumping wildly. I slid the cold instrument across her skin, pushing back the paper gown slightly, and there were more bruises, deep purple and yellowish brown. I didn't need a textbook to tell me these were old wounds. Or years of experience to confirm what my gut was telling me. I'd seen this kind of damage before . . . and not just in a hospital. My mother's face flashed through my mind. I took a deep breath and exhaled slowly. This would not be an easy conversation.

"Debra," I said quietly, recalling the name on her chart, "do you want to tell me again what happened?"

She just lay there silently at first, tears spilling from the corners of her eyes. She shook her head.

"It's okay," I said, trying to comfort her. "You can trust me. There are services that will help you. I can call a social worker, or the hospital's domestic violence hotline."

She shook her head even more vigorously—no!

But I kept pushing. "I can phone the Newark police and get someone here to protect you."

Suddenly she was emphatic: "I said no! Just fix me and let me go!"

The silence that followed was tense. "Will you be okay to go home?" I asked. "Is it safe?"

She nodded, but I knew otherwise. I'd spent much of my childhood tiptoeing around the land mines just beneath the surface of a volatile home—hearing, watching, my parents fight, sometimes violently. As hard as I always tried to respect my patients' wishes, I couldn't stop myself from prying, from trying to persuade Debra to let me help. The next questions just tumbled from my mouth:

"Why? Why are you protecting a man who hurts you?"

For the first time, Debra looked me squarely in the eyes, and I saw a toughness in her that I had not seen before: "Because Terry loves me, Doctor, that's why."

Terry was her husband of many years—her high school sweet-heart, the man with whom she had shared half her young life. He had driven her to the hospital and now sat in the waiting room, probably looking like the perfect, patient husband. I imagined him there, fidgeting anxiously, feeling sorry for himself, wondering why his wife had made him lose his temper and do such a terrible thing to her.

Debra squeezed her eyes shut, sighed deeply, and her story flowed as freely as her tears. "He didn't mean to do it," she began, admitting the beating that had sent her flying across the room and into the corner of her dresser.

What a coward, I thought, feeling anger at him rising inside me. But I tried to keep a straight face and professional distance as Debra talked about their life together. He was a good provider, she said, but even with both their incomes, they struggled to make ends meet. Like any couple, they had disagreements, she contin-ued, and at times things got out of hand. But it was usually her fault, she added. She always seemed to push the wrong buttons in him.

"I know he has a temper, and he warns me," she said. "But I just keep pushing." Next time, she would keep her mouth shut, and everything would be fine.

As I examined Debra's wounds, I thought: *I know this couple.* I'd seen their kind of "love" my entire life, the kind that can swing violently from passion to pain with one wrong word. And even after all my years of medical training, I still had no more answers than I'd had as a boy, watching in fear as my mother and father cursed and clawed at each other.

I'm sure there must have been a time when Moms thought Pop hit her because she'd pushed him too far or talked too much. They would exchange blows one minute and talk sweetly to each other the next—or so said my older sister Fellease, who along with my other sister, Roselene, and two older brothers witnessed the worst of our parents' battles. By the time my younger brother, Carlton, and I came along, any sweetness that had existed between our parents had turned bitter.

The only glimpse of love that I remember happened when I was about eleven. My parents were taking a photo together. My mother's brother and sister were visiting from Cleveland over Labor Day weekend, and as my aunt Doretha snapped a photo, my uncle TJ and his wife stood to the side, and I saw my father take my mother's hand and pull her close. It was the first time I'd ever even seen them hold hands. I held every detail of that moment in my mind: Moms in her red shorts and cream-colored blouse and Pop in a Miami Beach–like floral print shirt and blue trousers. There for a split second I saw what looked like a happy couple.

Truth was, they had carved out two separate lives under the same roof by then and most times dropped even the pretense of cordiality. They slept in different rooms on opposite ends of our small two-bedroom house—Pop in the master bedroom on the second floor and Moms on a twin bed in the basement. Carlton and I shared a sofa bed next to her.

Most days, my parents went about their business with just the required exchanges between them—a word or two here and there about a needed repair around the house, money, groceries, or the children. But the potential for a blowup always made me tense whenever their paths crossed. I could see Moms seething and suck-ing her teeth the moment he entered the room.

"Ma, stop that," I'd say, annoyed that she seemed about to pro-voke him into a fight.

Pop just walked around, mostly silent and withdrawn. One wrong word hurled in the other's direction at the wrong time, though, and the sparks began to fly.

"You crazy, bitch," Pop would shout.

"Well, you ain't shit," Moms would yell back.

I'd stand there speechless, praying that Moms would just be quiet or that Pop would walk away. At times, I felt like a pawn in their chess game, pushed this way or that in their effort to one-up the other, like the times when I'd run to my dad's side as a kid and plead with him to let me help work on the car or mow the lawn. I'd tug on his pants leg until he gave in. But the moment he let me join him, Moms quickly appeared and yelled for me. I was too little, or I was going to get hurt, she'd say, ordering me back inside. She made it clear that she didn't trust my father to keep me safe, but it seemed clear to me that she also didn't want me getting too close to him, lest he gain some kind of advantage in their war. As a child, I wanted to be just like my father and felt robbed of those stolen moments to learn manly things from him. Other times, I'd stand silently and hang my head as Pop berated my mother in my presence, trying to sway me to his point of view.

Some days I'd hide out in the backyard in my own private spot: a pile of rocks on a dirt patch next to the garage. I'd sit there, out of everyone's sight, and flip over the biggest stones and watch qui-etly as the community of worms that lived underneath scurried for cover. I'd lose myself in their quiet world. Mine seemed so tumul-tuous, and I always worried about what *could* happen—a fear branded into my soul by an unforgettable moment during the Christmas holidays when I was about six years old.

My mother and sisters were in the kitchen, preparing our traditional holiday feast, and Carlton, Andre, and I played nearby. The smooth baritone of Nat King Cole—one of Pop's favorites—rose from the stereo and floated throughout the house. Moms made her way to the living room, where Pop sat playing his beloved guitar to one of the Christmas classics.

"Turn that noise down," Moms ordered.

Pop had been drinking and stood his ground: "No, I will not!"

But my mother was never the type to back down, even when Pop tried to walk away. Whatever was on her mind came flying out of her mouth, like kindling thrown onto a heap of smoking hot debris. "Oh, yes, you will!"

Their ensuing argument sounded like familiar background noise—until things took a sudden and unexpected turn. Pop dashed up the stairs to his bedroom, where most times he would have stayed. But the next thing I knew, he was standing on the third step of the living room staircase with a gun pointed at the person I loved most in the world. Before that moment, I never even knew he had a gun.

"I'll shoot you, woman," he warned. "I will kill you!"

Moms shouted back with her typical fearlessness: "Go ahead. Shoot me."

This can't be happening . . . Please, God, don't let him do it, I prayed, too shocked even to cry. Carlton immediately began wailing. My sisters jumped from their chairs and stood in the middle of the battle, as if they could stop a flying bullet with their outstretched arms. Then, suddenly, Andre leaped up and yelled at our parents: "Why don't y'all stop!"

Maybe seeing the hurt he was causing his children got to Pop that day. He would never have intentionally hurt us. Without a word, he lowered the gun, climbed the stairs, and returned to hibernation in his room.

———

"Do the two of you have children?" I asked Debra during the examination.

Yes, she responded, their son was ten, and their daughter was eight. *Poor children,* I thought. They were bound to have witnessed their parents' battles, and there are few things more terrifying to a child. You feel helpless—and worse, somehow to blame. The guilt always comes, especially when the battles are about money. With a kid's sense of reasoning, you find yourself thinking that maybe your parents wouldn't fight so much if you weren't around, if you didn't need food, clothes, or a new pair of shoes. Every battle leaves a scar. Every fight alters a child's sense of what's normal. Down the road, some children who grew up with domestic violence rail against it, vowing—as I did—never to live like that. I even promised myself that I would never get married.

Many studies show that children who witness domestic violence are more likely than other children to become abusers or victims of abuse themselves. In such cases, fighting is seen as a normal part of living and loving. Girls who saw a parent abused often choose boyfriends or husbands who beat them; the women accept it because they expect it. Likewise, the boys frequently become batterers who see their version of manhood as the real way to keep a loudmouthed, strong-willed woman in check.

I pleaded with Debra: Think of your children and the unhealthy environment they are living in. Get help for them, if not for yourself, I warned. But her eyes narrowed, fairly screaming that this was none of my business. I knew then that I'd stepped across a line. I'd violated that unspoken urban creed I'd learned back on Dayton Street: Whatever happens between a man and his woman is nobody else's business.

Not here, though, I thought. *Not in my shop. Not anymore.*

"I'm bound by law to report to authorities if I suspect a crime has been committed," I told Debra. I was still so green that I had no idea whether this was even true. I'd learn later that the law requires only that I report cases of homicide, weapons injuries, or suspected elder or child abuse, and that I had no real grounds to report Debra. But I was willing to bluff if it meant I could possibly save her life.

"No, Dr. Davis! If you call the cops, Terry will get in trouble," she replied.

He was on probation, she said, and she needed him at home to help raise their children.

"Besides," she added, "I hit him sometimes, too."

Debra didn't see herself as a victim, because she fought back. And as many desperate women do, she had decided she couldn't make it without her man's financial support. Most domestic violence victims—upward of 95 percent—are women, and the vast majority of them never leave their abusers. Just 30 percent ever even seek help for their injuries in an emergency room.

This was my chance to do something. I couldn't just stitch up Debra's face and send her back to the man whose fists had landed her in my care in the first place.

I sat on the doctor stool in room A4, working quietly. Suddenly, I was a tough, curly-haired ten-year-old boy again, back on Dayton Street one sweltering summer day in 1983. My boys and I had just finished a game of Twenty-one in street basketball and had walked over to the hot dog truck that was a permanent fixture in the neighborhood. We called it "the hot dog truck," but it was actually a van, stocked with everything from hot dogs and chips to penny candies, sodas, and juices. You could buy something there with any coin you pulled from your pocket. Maybe I would get lucky enough to find a quarter to buy some juice. As I stood there, dressed in my blue basketball shorts, white T-shirt, and PRO-Keds sneakers, I dug into my pockets. My eyes fell on a thermometer attached to a utility pole a few inches away. It registered 102 degrees. No wonder I'd felt so beaten down after pulling off the basketball victory—scoring the twenty-one points before anyone else. My mouth felt parched, and as I finally found the quarter and pulled it out of my pocket, I felt like I had won the lottery.

"Gimme a grape," I said, asking the vendor for my favorite.

I stuck my sweaty face inside the van, hoping to feel a bit of the frost rising from the freezer as the man opened it to hand me my prize. Suddenly, a loud commotion from the high-rise public housing projects across Ludlow Street caught my attention. People were gathering around Building 6. There were screams, the instant wail of sirens, and flashes of red, blue, and orange lights from police cars that screeched to a halt in a gigantic dirt patch that was once a grassy play area just past the projects. Police cars blocked off my street. A uniformed officer ran past me with his gun drawn, heading in the direction of the commotion. More officers followed, racing to the scene in their bulletproof vests. Some had rifles. In my neighborhood, I was accustomed to sirens and flashing lights at all hours, but this much police action meant something tragic had occurred. My first thought was to wonder whether someone I knew had died. Still holding my juice, I sprinted with my boys to the scene.

As we arrived, an officer was using the familiar yellow tape to block off the building. He instructed the crowd to back up. Since my friends and I were small, we managed to snake our way to the front. Neighbors seemed to come from all directions, until there were probably a hundred sweaty bodies gathered behind the tape. We all just stood there, waiting, and watching the police officers' every move, like spectators at a game. Before long, a black station wagon pulled up and slowly made its way directly in front of Building 6. An obese middle-aged white man in a frumpy suit hopped out and wobbled to the building's entrance. A half hour or so later, the man reappeared, with a group of police officers pushing a stretcher carrying a black body bag. A collective gasp rose from the crowd at the sight of it. I felt a familiar knot in the pit of my stomach. Somebody had died for sure, and more likely than not, it was someone we knew. The officers lifted the stretcher and rolled it into the back of the station wagon. The crowd speculated loudly about what might have happened. Had a drug deal gone bad? Had a rival gang member stepped onto the wrong turf? But the puzzle pieces fell quickly into place when police officers brought out their handcuffed assailant.

"Oh my God, Brenda!" a woman in the crowd shrieked.

Another collective gasp went up.

Even us younger ones could figure this out. The person in the body bag must have been Brenda's husband, Dave. Everybody either knew the couple or knew about them. They were quite a pair—ideal during the week, always together, laughing and talking with neighbors outside in the common areas, grocery shopping, strolling along the sidewalks. But they drank on weekends, and their sixth-floor apartment became their battleground. In the summer, the yelling, screaming, and sounds of breaking glass would travel down through their open windows, to the walkways and playgrounds below. *Brenda and Dave are at it again,* someone would say, as if that was a normal part of life and love. Sometimes, the couple would go after each other outdoors, in full view of anyone who happened to be watching. They'd curse each other out, throw punches, and occasionally even pull out a knife.

"Y'all need to take that indoors," one of the adults might yell, out of respect for us children, watching in amusement.

Sometimes police would get an anonymous call, and we'd see Dave led away in handcuffs. He would disappear for a week or two, but they always made their way back to each other. Privately,

Brenda's friends—including my sister Fellease—urged her to leave him. But even when Brenda got enough nerve to do so, she didn't stay away. Dave showered her with gifts, money, flowers, and notes telling her he couldn't live without her.

Just one year earlier, it had been Brenda brought out on a gurney by emergency medical personnel after they'd had a horrendous fight. I could hardly believe my eyes when I saw her bloody, swollen face with large, open wounds, which made her look like she'd been mauled by a pit bull. It appeared as though Dave had bitten or clawed chunks out of her face. Brenda was hospitalized for weeks. When she got out, she confided in Fellease that Dave had called her daily from jail, crying and pleading for her forgiveness. He didn't know what came over him when he drank, he said. He would stop drinking and never hit her again. He promised. She was beautiful, he told her, and the two of them were made for each other.

Brenda held out longer than anyone expected, but she eventually refused to testify against Dave, and the charges were dropped. Dave was released, and as usual, the couple reconciled. All of us who were her neighbors and friends thought Brenda was crazy for returning to him, and I'm sure Fellease told her so. But it didn't matter to Brenda what anyone else thought of Dave. He had persuaded her that no one would love her more than he did. And as her once-attractive face began to show her battle scars, she actually believed that no one but Dave *could* ever love her. When she went back to him that time, though, she quietly bought a gun— just in case she needed to protect herself, she told Fellease. For a while, Dave held true to his word. He quit drinking. To everyone's surprise, nearly a year passed without any public fights between the couple, and there was no yelling or screaming from their sixth-floor window. Even my sister was beginning to believe that Dave was indeed a changed man.

But on that stifling summer day as my boys and I played a game of Twenty-one, Brenda and Dave were at it again, a few of the neighbors later told me. They heard Dave cursing, and Brenda screaming for him to stop. There were loud bumps against the walls. Things seemed to settle down for a bit, the neighbors said, but a half hour later, two loud pops rang out. They sounded like firecrackers. Then came the police, the crowd, and the body bag.

"Dr. Davis," Debra said, interrupting my thoughts and breaking the long silence between us in room A4, "if you're done, then I'm ready to go."

Her husband was waiting, she said, and they needed to get home to their children.

Debra's face had required twenty-five stitches. Long suture procedures were part of the grunt work for first-year residents. I had never done that many stitches on one patient before, so my neat work gave me a momentary sense of pride. But I wasn't finished just yet.

"Debra," I said, looking her straight in her eyes, "I've seen people die in relationships like this. Your husband needs help, and so do you."

"Dr. Davis, I know Terry has his problems, but—"

"Next time," I said, interrupting her, "he may kill you."

But like a woman resigned to her fate, Debra answered solemnly: "I'll have to cross that bridge when I come to it."

I could tell those were her final words. Nothing I'd said had reached her. She was planning to leave the hospital with her attacker, and I could do nothing about it. Then, for some inexplicable reason, I just gave up. Maybe nothing I said or did would have made a difference that day. But maybe with more experience, I would have had the confidence to ignore her pleas, to call the domestic violence hotline, to report the incident to the police. It was a thought that would haunt me for years. In that moment, though, when a split-second decision was required, I couldn't think of anything more persuasive to say.

"Okay, Debra," I responded, and then recited by rote the standard spiel for care of her wounds. "You need a wound check in forty-eight hours, and the sutures need to come out in five to seven days. If the wounds become red or start to leak pus, or if you develop a fever, come back right away. You'll have scars from your injuries."

And I wasn't just talking about facial scars.

As I prepared to leave the room, I jotted down my number at the hospital and handed it to her. "If you ever need help or just want to talk, give me a call," I told her.

Debra thanked me, but I knew she would never call. Moms had never called anyone for help either. She always figured she could handle my father. I guess it's fortunate that the worst damage they ever caused each other were bruises and a few nasty cuts. But I spent an inordinate amount of my childhood worrying that one of them would wind up in a cemetery and the other in jail for murder. I prayed Debra's case wouldn't end that way. One in five domestic abuse cases does, I knew, and usually the victim is the one killed. All I was absolutely sure of was this: Debra's husband would beat her again.

Debra was still on my mind when I headed home early the next morning after my twelve-hour shift. I lay awake for hours, as I often did, wrestling with what I could have said or should have done differently. I knew it in my heart: *I shouldn't have let her go.*

My mind wound back to Brenda and Dave. For the longest time after Brenda went to jail, I wondered what had gone so wrong between the two of them that final time. Why couldn't they have just stayed away from each other? I'd wondered the same about my parents. In some ways it was a relief when my father finally left for good when I was twelve. At least the fights stopped.

It didn't occur to me till much later, though, what I'd missed by rarely seeing happily married couples. I can't recall seeing, on a regular basis, any examples of romantic love that didn't involve a great deal of suffering and pain. Even the few couples I knew who had somehow managed to stay together seemed more committed to some ideal of long-suffering than to each other's happiness; whatever joy they might have once found together seemed long gone. The kind of love and relationships I saw in the movies and on *The Cosby Show* seemed about as fake and unattainable to me as the middle-class lives of the characters. *Yeah, right,* I thought to myself after yet another episode of my favorite TV show wrapped up neatly with Clair and Heathcliff Huxtable—a lawyer and a doctor—still loving each other after whatever challenge they'd faced. *Yeah, right,* I thought again, secretly wishing I was one of those lucky children.

But even though I desired the success, status, and peaceful life of the Huxtables, I could hardly imagine that life. I must have been a teenager when I first told myself that I would never go through the hell of marriage or put anyone else through it. I'd felt the racing heart, sweaty hands, shot-to-the-loins kind of feelings. That wasn't hard to understand. It was what came next that puzzled me. What was a couple to do once the excitement of just being together wore off? How were two individuals supposed to negotiate the differences that inevitably became apparent? How could each one maintain his or her individuality without the other feeling threatened? I had no blueprint for any of it. I've always wanted to be good at everything I did, even when I was hustling. And nothing in my experience had me believing it was possible to have a truly happy marriage—one that was still happy when the door shut to the outside world.

I was in college the first time I told a girl "I love you" and really believed I meant it. But even then, I wasn't comfortable opening my heart completely—it seemed to give her too much power. The more I opened up my life to her, the more vulnerable I felt. A real man just didn't do that, or so I thought. What if she hurt me? Would I become the kind of coward who needed to beat his woman into submission to feel powerful? This question stayed in the back of my mind, and I challenged myself to learn from what I'd seen. I had no vision of the kind of man I wanted to be; I just knew I didn't want to repeat the behavior I had witnessed. I promised myself from the time I started dating that I would never hit a woman. Somehow, I would be better, stronger, I told myself.

But getting there took time. It took unlearning the lessons of my childhood.

In high school, I sometimes behaved badly, treating girls like they were as dispensable as clothes, trying different ones, leaving behind a trail of tears and heartbreak. That had me feeling empty, but it seemed better than the alternative. At least that way, I thought foolishly, I maintained my manhood. I was in control.

In my senior year of college, though, I fell hard.

I had been accepted into a new program for minority students, Access-Med, a joint venture between Rutgers University and the Robert Wood Johnson Medical School. The program offered the chance for me to get some of my first-year medical school courses out of the way by taking them in my senior year of college. That would ensure a lighter load in my first year of medical school—an intensive period when many overwhelmed students drop out. It also would guarantee acceptance (depending, of course, on my academic performance) into Robert Wood Johnson without having to take the MCAT, the standardized test usually required to enter medical school. I transferred from Seton Hall University to Rutgers to complete my senior year of college and to participate in the program. There I met my girl in the cafeteria of the university's Livingston campus. When I first saw her, I couldn't take my eyes off her. She was fine—petite with pecan-colored skin and narrow deep brown eyes. The two of us clicked immediately and quickly became inseparable as a couple. She was different from the fast party girls I often met. She was sweet and nurturing but not the least bit boring. She knew how to have a good time at a party, but she was just as comfortable staying at home. She was confident and didn't waver on the things in life she wanted. I loved that about her, but after about two years of dating, her decisiveness—or she might say, my indecisiveness—began to cause problems for us. She wanted to settle down and get married. I wasn't ready. Aside from my ambivalence about marriage, I was in my second year of medical school, and my studies were demanding more of my time. It seemed to her that I was pulling away. She wasn't going to compete with my career for my attention, she said. She called things off.

On impulse one Friday night, I decided I needed to see her— right then. It had been about a week since we broke up, and I was missing her badly. Maybe we could talk and work things out, I reasoned. I didn't want to give her a chance to say no, so I showed up at her dorm room unannounced. I knew her roommate usually went home on weekends, so my girl had the place all to herself. The main doors to the dorm stayed locked at night, but I was certain I could get inside the way I had many times before when I visited her after hours: I would wait around outside and follow one of the residents in. My plan worked. I dashed up the stairs to her second-floor room and instinctively turned the doorknob. It wasn't locked, which meant she was probably in the shower. I had warned her many times about leaving the door unlocked, even while she walked down the hall to the bathroom. I stepped inside her room to wait and surprise her. The anticipation of that sweet moment gave me a rush. She would run into my arms, wearing nothing but her robe, smelling fresh with the light, flowery scent of her favorite body wash. We'd kiss, tell each other how lonely we'd been, and she'd ask me to spend the night with her.

Her room was dark, but not completely. And what I made out startled me. Someone—not her, the body frame was too large— was asleep in her bed, and the covers were pulled over the mystery person's face. My eyes turned to a pair of worn boots and denim jeans lying on the floor beside the bed. Damn, it was a dude. She'd already invited another man into her bed? My heart and mind quickly filled with rage. What should I do? Kick him out that moment? Wait and confront her? I felt the urge to rush down the hall, grab her out of the shower, and demand some answers.

As I stood there quietly for a moment, still in shock, contemplating my next move, I felt the veins pulse in my head. I exited the room as quietly as I had entered it and squatted around the corner. I had a full view of her door, but she wouldn't see me. The shower in the community bathroom stopped, and I knew she was just moments from walking out.

My head hurt, and the rage inside me only grew as I saw her, as beautiful as ever, strolling down the hallway in her robe and slippers. She was supposed to be as heartsick as I was over our breakup, unable to eat or sleep. What was she planning to do when she got to the room? Did she have anything on under that robe? Why were his jeans off? Was she going to make love to him? Had they made love already? It had been only a week since we'd ended things. One week! We were in love. She had told me she loved me. And I loved her. Had she played me? The beast inside me was rattling the cage. And I felt the urge to punish her, hurt her the way I was hurting.

So, this is how it happens, I thought, feeling justified in my fury. *This is how it all goes down.* Before I could figure out what to do or say, she was entering her room. I rushed from my hiding place, grabbed the door before she could close it behind her, and followed her inside. Startled at the sight of me, she jumped back and ran to her roommate's side of the room. I saw terror in her eyes, but I wanted her to be afraid, to hurt, and to feel my hurt. She deserved whatever happened for hurting me this way. I walked over to her bed and snatched the covers off the guy. He had three seconds to get his stuff, or it was going to be down, I warned. Jeans and boots in hand, he fled the room. The coward didn't even have the guts to stick around, I taunted. As I walked toward her, I noticed she was crying. I saw a reflection of myself in her frightened eyes. It unnerved me. What was I doing? But the beast wouldn't let me back down. *She* had hurt *me*. I walked toward her with my hand balled into a fist, my rage boiling. I unleashed it all with a powerful punch. I'd intentionally struck the wall.

"How could you?" I yelled.

My fist trembled from the impact.

"How could you?"

I stared at the floor for what felt like forever. I could give in to the rage that was threatening to take control of me. Or I could walk away. I chose the latter. While I'm not proud of how close I came to losing control, I learned that day that I was strong enough to reject the kind of violence I'd seen during my life.

Unfortunately, dating violence is far too prevalent among college students. In a 2011 survey commissioned by Liz Claiborne Inc. as part of its "Love Is Not Abuse" program, 43 percent of college women reported having experienced abusive behaviors while dating. That includes physical, sexual, or verbal abuse, or the use of digital technology in an abusive manner, like the guy who constantly checks his girlfriend's emails and text messages or demands that she delete certain friends from her Facebook list. Also, 52 percent of the college women surveyed said they had a friend who'd experienced such abusive behaviors, and nearly one in three reported having been involved in an actual abusive relationship.

In addition to the survey, which included 508 college students, Liz Claiborne Inc. put together a task force of educators and domestic violence experts from various universities, who came up with a curriculum that teaches students about the dangers and warning signs of dating abuse, offers lessons on avoiding and protecting yourself from the increased use of technology to harass and abuse, and provides resources for students to find help. The task force was created after the highly publicized murder of Yeardley Love, a twenty-two-year-old University of Virginia lacrosse player, in May 2010. Love's on-and-off boyfriend, George W. Huguely, a fellow University of Virginia student and lacrosse player, was convicted of second-degree murder and sentenced to twenty-three years in prison. Huguely was drunk when he kicked his way through the door to her bedroom and wrestled her to the floor after she refused to talk to him. He admitted shaking her and slamming her head against a wall. He then left her to die on a blood-soaked pillow. On the way out, he stole her computer. She was discovered hours later by her horrified roommate.

Courtroom testimony portrayed Huguely as a possessive, controlling boyfriend who sent Love a threatening email just days before their final night together. He'd heard that she'd been romantically linked to a lacrosse player from a rival school, and he fired off a message that said, in part: "I should have killed you."

These were young people of privilege, unlike the young men and women I most often encounter in the emergency room. But rich or poor, domestic abuse and dating violence hurt the same.

Nearly two years after my encounter with Debra in the emergency room, I was wrapping up a thirty-hour shift at University Hospital when I noticed the on-duty trauma team working furiously on a female patient. She was limp on a stretcher in a corner of the department. I immediately ripped off my jacket, ran toward my co-workers, and gloved up. The patient needed intravenous access to deliver lifesaving fluids and medications to her depleted body. I grabbed the triple lumen catheter and placed a large bore needle in her chest through the vein known as the subclavian. This advanced procedure requires quick, smooth hands to guide the needle in the right direction. Aiming it directly under the collarbone, I had to be careful not to puncture the patient's lungs. During the procedure, I quickly eyeballed her. She had multiple bruises, ranging from deep brown to yellow and green, indicating she'd been beaten over a period of days . . . and beaten badly. Maybe she had been held hostage, I thought.

She had a weak pulse, and her blood pressure was dropping. No doubt she was bleeding internally. With the central line in place, she was finally receiving the needed fluids. The anesthesiologist completed the intubation. The patient was holding on.

I walked to the head of the bed and noticed a well-healed facial scar over her eyebrow. It jogged my memory. I'd taken care of this woman before, but where? The more I looked at her bloody, beaten face, the more familiar she looked. I quickly went to the nursing station and grabbed her chart. My exhausted eyes scanned it, looking for her name. There it was: Mrs. Debra Cooper. Debra. The same Debra. I stood there in shock, her blood on my gloves and scrubs. I knew right away who had done this to her. Again. She'd insisted on staying with her husband, despite my warnings. But I was full of regret. *I should have called the police,* I thought. Just then, a nurse grabbed my elbow.

"Dr. Davis, you're needed in the trauma bay," she said.

I hurried back to the room and joined the team. Debra had lost her pulse and was in traumatic cardiac arrest. I began chest compressions. She had suffered severe blunt trauma to her head, chest, and abdomen. We worked for another thirty minutes, delivering all sorts of interventions, but nothing worked. We couldn't bring her back. I pronounced Debra dead at 11:30 A.M.

On average, more than three women are murdered by their husband or boyfriend every day. With Debra's death, one more woman who'd remained in an abusive relationship was gone forever. The children she'd stayed to protect were without their mother. And those of us who could have called for help are left to wonder: What if?

Does Your Partner

- Embarrass you with put-downs?
- Look at you or act in ways that scare you?
- Control what you do, whom you see or talk to, or where you go?
- Stop you from seeing your friends or family members?
- Take your money or Social Security check, make you ask for money, or refuse to give you money?
- Make all of the decisions?
- Tell you that you're a bad parent or threaten to take away or hurt your children?
- Prevent you from working or attending school?
- Act like the abuse is no big deal, it's your fault, or even deny abusing you?
- Destroy your property or threaten to kill your pets?
- Intimidate you with guns, knives, or other weapons?
- Shove you, slap you, choke you, or hit you?
- Force you to try to drop charges?
- Threaten to commit suicide?
- Threaten to kill you?

IF YOU ANSWERED "YES" TO EVEN ONE OF THESE QUESTIONS, YOU MAY BE IN AN ABUSIVE RELATIONSHIP.

For support and more information, call the National Domestic Violence Hotline at:

1-800-799-SAFE (7233) or TTY 1-800-787-3224

Source: The National Domestic Violence Hotline

5

DYING FOR LOVE

By my second year of residency, I'd begun to notice a disturbing pattern on the A side: During practically every shift, I was diagnosing or treating at least one patient with a sexually transmitted infection. Gonorrhea. Syphilis. Genital warts. Chlamydia. Herpes. And more.

One day I knocked on A3 and entered to find an attractive twenty-five-year-old woman named Danielle. She looked so serene sitting on the examining room table in a bright yellow hospital gown. Her almond-colored face wore a slight smile. Her chart told me part of the story. The rest was left to her mother, Mary Rogers, a chatty, dignified woman who appeared to be in her late fifties. Mrs. Rogers was a retired fourth grade teacher who had worked thirty years in the school system before leaving the classroom to take care of her only child.

"Dr. Davis, I love children," Mrs. Rogers said soon after our introductions. "I told Danielle to get married and have as many as possible."

A flash of pain crossed the mother's face. She stared longingly at her daughter, a younger version of herself, sitting a few feet away, wearing a sweet, clueless smile. Danielle no longer remembered the life she once had. She'd forgotten her job as an assistant communications specialist in the U.S. Army. She'd forgotten her many friends, her apartment address, and her cell phone number. She'd even forgotten the love of her life, the man who'd infected her with genital herpes. When the symptoms appeared, Danielle must have been terrified—so terrified that she didn't go to the doctor right away. That allowed the virus to progress into a rare, aggressive form called "herpes encephalitis," which had invaded her brain and destroyed the cells responsible for behavior and memory. By the time Danielle finally sought help, the virus had already begun the destruction that would leave her with the mental capacity of a child, and the damage was irreversible. Mary Rogers had dedicated herself to serving not only as her daughter's caretaker but as her living, breathing scrapbook.

"Danielle was an ambitious, outgoing young lady with a bright future," Mrs. Rogers said, suddenly beaming. "She was employee of the month three separate times. She led Bible study every Saturday morning. She only missed one Saturday, and that was to come be with me after I had surgery."

It seemed important to Mrs. Rogers that I knew her daughter had been a good girl, that she hadn't always been sick. I nodded and smiled, trying to imagine the vibrant young woman Danielle used to be, but I could think only of what this tragedy had wrought. The nervous system, including the brain, is the body's hard drive, and damage to it can quickly shut down primary functions, like walking, talking, or thinking. The damage is often debilitating and permanent. For Danielle, there would be no more nights out with the girls, no more job promotions, no wedding, no children. She would have to live the rest of her days trapped in childhood, without the innocence, the fun, or the hope. Unprotected sex had cost her much of her future and had altered her mother's life as well. If only Danielle had protected herself, if only she had gone to a doctor when the first blisters and swelling appeared, but it was too late for that now. All I could do was treat the symptoms that had brought her to the emergency room that afternoon. I glanced down at the form the triage nurse had prepared and asked Mrs. Rogers about Danielle's fever.

"She felt warm to me," her mother said. "And when I took her temperature, it was high. Her doctor always told me to bring Danielle to the hospital if she has a fever or isn't acting her normal self. Since her disease, she isn't as reliable with how she feels. Most of the time, I have to guess what's wrong with her . . . Danielle used to be so independent. Even as a child she wanted to find her own way. I remember she would pick out her clothes for daycare when she was three. She always wanted to wear her pink rubber boots, with any outfit at all."

As with my pediatric cases, I had to rely fully on Mrs. Rogers's description of Danielle's symptoms to come up with a game plan. The fever had lasted a couple of days so far, and Danielle, who didn't eat much on a normal day, now ate nothing at all.

I kept probing: "Anything else going on—any vomiting, diarrhea, cough, congestion?"

"Well, she has been pointing to her bladder area, saying it burns," Mrs. Rogers said. "I've noticed she moans when she goes to the bathroom. There also seems to be a strange smell to her urine, which is new."

It sounded like a bladder infection. I explained to Mrs. Rogers that I was ordering blood work and a urine sample to be sure. Usually, that would have been my signal to move on to the next patient. In emergency medicine, there's little time to linger, because a new crisis is always waiting. But I pushed aside the hurried feeling in my gut and stood there, in awe of this mother's dedication. I sensed, too, that she needed a sympathetic, non-judgmental ear.

Doctors had recommended an assisted living center for Danielle, Mrs. Rogers said. But no way would she put her baby girl in some wretched place, where people might not take care of her. Mrs. Rogers reminded me a bit of my own mother, who had been protective in that way, too, when my older sister Fellease got sick.

I was in college when I figured out Fellease had AIDS. Back then, the early nineties, it was still largely viewed among African Americans as a gay white man's disease (even though the statistics were beginning to tell another story), and there were plenty of examples in the news of victims who were ostracized and mistreated. The not-so-subtle message was: If you had AIDS or knew someone who did, you didn't talk about it. But turning her back on anyone in a crisis has never been part of my mother's makeup, especially not her own flesh and blood.

Once, when growing up, I counted fourteen people living under our roof, that small two-bedroom house with just one and a half bathrooms. All around me were sisters, brothers, nieces, nephews, uncles, cousins, in-laws, and close friends, all struggling in some way—either through unemployment, marital issues, drug addiction, or alcoholism—and in need of a place to stay until they could get on their feet. At night, I'd see Moms tossing pillows and bed linens into every open space in the house, even the dining room. Likewise, she ignored relatives or friends who wondered aloud whether you could catch "the AIDS" from a toilet seat or a clean spoon or fork that hadn't been sterilized in bleach. Her baby girl was welcome, sick or not, and if people had a problem with that, they need not visit.

Fel was a crack addict who moved from place to place, but Moms cooked for her every day, in case my sister swooped in and wanted to eat. Moms also knew right away who the culprit was when things of value suddenly began disappearing from the house. Though my mother fussed and cussed about it, she never shut her doors to her child. I'd see the worry all over Moms's face when Fel mysteriously disappeared for days at a time.

As for me, I worried about my mother almost as much as I did about my big sister. And it was Moms's strain I saw in Mrs. Rogers's face. The puffy, dark circles underneath her eyes announced clearly that she wasn't getting enough rest.

"Mrs. Rogers, all this must be hard for you," I said, acknowledging that I saw her suffering, too. She nodded, and tears pooled in her eyes.

"She was in love," Mrs. Rogers said, as though she could still hardly believe it all. "The boyfriend left as soon as he realized what happened. I called his family, but there wasn't much I could do."

Her daughter had been planning to wear her mother's wedding gown when she walked down the aisle. "If her father was alive today, I know Eddie would beat that boy's behind," Mrs. Rogers said. "Look at my poor baby. Never did I plan on this. What mother could plan for this?"

I absorbed her heartbreaking words, letting her talk.

Danielle had been a military brat. The family had traveled the world with Eddie, who'd been a soldier in the U.S. Army. "She wanted to be just like her daddy. That's all she talked about," Mrs. Rogers said.

Danielle loved the uniforms, the stripes, the decorum of the army, and as early as high school, she began mapping out a plan for her military future. She enlisted right after her high school graduation, determined to make a career in the U.S. Army, and was well on her way. Sadness and resignation seemed to settle on the mother's face when she got to this part of the story. It wasn't supposed to end there. Mrs. Rogers grew quiet.

"I'm so sorry about what happened to your daughter," I said.

She thanked me. I handed her the urine cup and pointed the way to the bathroom. "The nurse will be in when you get back."

Within an hour, I had the test results and returned to the room to talk to Mrs. Rogers. Danielle indeed had a bladder infection, I told her. I explained that I was prescribing a regimen of antibiotics that Danielle would have to take twice a day for seven days, but that the two of them should follow up with Danielle's doctor. The mother seemed relieved by the diagnosis; at least her daughter would soon be out of this particular misery. I wished I could have done more than just treat the bladder infection, but the damage had already been done.

No way should Mrs. Rogers have been taking care of her daughter a second time around. While herpes encephalitis is extremely rare, it can be devastating to those it attacks. I wished in that moment that I could show Danielle's face and share her story with every young lady out there making bad decisions about sex, often in an empty quest for love and validation—especially African Americans. They're not the only ones having unprotected sex, of course, or the only ones contracting sexually transmitted infections. But the prevalence of these diseases among black women has been disproportionately high.

Educators report that sexual activity, from oral sex to intercourse, is beginning as early as middle school. My guess is that African American females are no more promiscuous than their peers of other races, but they do, unfortunately, have less access to good healthcare—nearly one-fifth of African Americans have no health insurance, statistics show—sex education, and reliable information, and thus are suffering more.

A study conducted by Dr. Sami Gottlieb, M.D., at the University of Colorado in Denver, showed in the mid-1990s that African American women were at a higher risk than any other group for infection with herpes simplex virus type 2, the most common type of herpes. It was one of the largest studies of its kind, involving questionnaires and blood tests from more than 4,000 people who visited STI clinics in five cities, including Newark, between July 1993 and September 1996.

Most times, when I asked the young women I treated why they didn't insist on a condom, they said they thought they could trust their partner. It never seemed to occur to them that their partner might not have known he was infected—or worse, just didn't care. I've seen that, too, like the two teenage boys who showed up in the E.R. together one evening for treatment. Both were experiencing penile discharge, and they laughed when I told them they had contracted an STI from their sexual encounter—presumably, from their banter, the same girl. There seemed to be a weird man-code thing going on, because they asked to be treated together. Then, as if it was some kind of honor, they smacked each other high fives when the nurse appeared with a needle and syringe to administer the antibiotic. I told them their partner needed to be notified so she could be treated, too, but they shrugged it off. Their response angered me.

"What if this was your mother or sister?" I asked, hoping that might get through to them.

Smirking, one of the teens responded: "Please, Doc. That ain't my problem."

I thought of my own sister and felt a strong urge to smack both of them. I left the room wanting to run to the hospital rooftop with a megaphone, yelling to the young women in my community: "Take control of your own sexuality! Protect yourselves! You're suffering, dying needlessly!"

Surveillance reports from the Centers for Disease Control and Prevention show significant racial disparities in the rates of sexually transmitted infections. It is worth noting that the source of the CDC's data is local and state health departments, which tend to base their reports on information from public health clinics. Since such clinics are used more often by minorities than whites, the differences in rates may be skewed. But other population-based surveys also confirm striking racial disparities. The point is, there's much work to do in convincing young men and women of color that this is a crisis that doesn't have to be, that they have the power to protect themselves and their partners. Here are the facts:

- In 2010, the rate of chlamydia among black females ages fifteen to nineteen was nearly seven times the rate of white females in the same age group; the rate among black women ages twenty to twenty-four was more than five times the rate of white women the same age; the rate among black males ages fifteen to nineteen was thirteen times that of their white peers; for black men ages twenty to twenty-four the rate was almost eight times that of white men the same age. Among Hispanics, the rate was three times that of whites; for Native Americans and Alaska natives, four times.
- In 2010, 69 percent of all reported cases of gonorrhea occurred among blacks. The rate of gonorrhea among blacks was nearly nineteen times that of whites. For black men, the rate was twenty-two times higher than that of their white peers; for black women, sixteen times. The rate among Hispanics was two times that of whites; for Native Americans and Alaska natives, nearly five times.
- In 2010, the rate of syphilis among black men was seven times the rate of white men; the rate among black women, twenty-one times that of white women. The rate for Hispanics was two times the rate for whites.
- Despite making up only about 14 percent of the U.S. population in 2009, African Americans accounted for 44 percent of new HIV infections that year.
- Compared with other races and ethnicities, African Americans account for a higher proportion of HIV infections at all stages of the disease—from new infections to deaths.

By the end of 2000, my sister Fellease's health had begun a rapid decline. I'd watched AIDS whittle her down from a robust 160 pounds to less than a hundred, mere skin and bones for a woman her height. She'd lost her teeth and developed vitiligo, white blotches like bleach stains all over her cinnamon-colored skin. Through it all, though, she never lost her zest for life—or her smile.

"I'm still pretty," she'd say, flashing that big, toothless grin at me, even as AIDS was ravaging her once beautiful face and frame. "We're twins."

Actually, fourteen years separated us. But of my five brothers and sisters, I was closest to her. I was the baby boy Fel never had. When I was growing up, she helped take care of me, bought me treats on demand, and talked the belt out of my parents' hands many times after I'd misbehaved. She was the cool big sister who kept me up on all the latest music and dances and even covered for me a time or two when I was hanging out somewhere I shouldn't have been. She always tried to tell me the right thing to do, even when we both knew she didn't make the best choices herself. When I heard the police were looking for me after I'd been involved with the robbery in my senior year of high school, I called Fel. Terrified that I'd probably just blown any shot at a real future, I anguished over whether I should turn myself in.

"We'll figure something out," Fel assured me. She drove me to the police station and talked mightily, trying to persuade the officers to release me into her care since I was a juvenile. Even though they took me into custody anyway, I never doubted that turning myself in that day was the right thing to do.

Fel had dropped out of high school to get married. She then divorced, remarried, and moved to Hawaii with her new husband, who was in the army. There she earned a high school equivalency diploma. Unfortunately, that marriage didn't last either. I was in the ninth grade when she returned to Newark, got a job, and lived at home on and off. The two of us grew even closer, staying up together many late nights, talking about life and playing board games.

But the streets had already started to claim her. In her room at our parents' house, I once discovered a burnt spoon and a tiny nip bottle of Bacardi rum that she had transformed into a crack pipe. I never told a soul, but it confirmed what I'd suspected: She was a crack addict. I just kept hoping she'd turn her life around, get a stable job again, find a great guy, have kids. Instead, she became more unreliable and unstable, moving from job to job, living here and there, and disappointing Moms and me again and again. When I discovered one day that money I'd been saving from my part-time job to repair my used car was missing from its hiding spot at home, I confronted Fel. She denied stealing it and denied using drugs, but I knew she was lying. Exasperated, I didn't speak to her for weeks.

Fel wasn't an IV drug user, but she was involved with men who were, and one of them undoubtedly infected her during sex. Maybe she didn't think her man needed to use a condom because she trusted him, as so many women claim. Or maybe, as an addict, she was just doing what it took to get the next high, and safety was the least of her concerns. But anytime you make the choice to practice unsafe sex, you're vulnerable; you're taking the risk of sharing whatever infections and diseases your partners and your partners' partners may have.

Fel didn't look sick right away; oddly, her hair texture was the first noticeable change. It became suddenly fine and silky. In the hood, the sudden emergence of "good hair" on a person with risky behaviors is suspect.

"She's got the package," we'd say, talking in code about one woman or another we suspected was infected with AIDS. Yet, despite the many times we said and heard that, it never occurred to us that AIDS had taken a deadly turn into urban communities. Poor black folks were dying at rates that nearly rivaled that of gay men when the disease first struck, and black women were being hit disproportionately hard. By 2001, AIDS had become the leading cause of death for African American women ages twenty-five to thirty-four, according to the Centers for Disease Control and Prevention, and most of them were being infected through sex with men who had been IV drug users or had sexual encounters with other men.

Fel denied my suspicion about her illness, just like she'd denied the theft and her drug use. I hinted one day that she had "that good hair," and she knew instantly what I meant. She snapped back that she didn't have "no HIV." But time revealed the truth. Back in the early 1990s, before drug cocktails made AIDS more of a terrible chronic illness than a death sentence, the virus killed slowly. Its victims had a certain look: emaciated bodies, sunken eyes, and sometimes even distinctive lesions. They were like walking ghosts with the dreaded "A" on their foreheads. In medical school, I'd fantasized about finding a cure. I wanted to save my sister, and it hurt deeply that I couldn't.

Just three months after I began my residency at Beth Israel, Fel started showing up in the E.R. with various AIDS-related ailments. She was loud and brash, demanding that the hospital staff bring Dr. Davis, her little brother, to her side. My colleagues thought it was a joke, that she was just another patient from the neighborhood claiming to be related to me to get quicker service, which sometimes happened. *Surely,* I could practically hear them thinking, *Dr. Davis doesn't have a sister like that.* For most of the doctors and nurses, Newark was just where they worked. But for me, it was home, and *those people* were my mother, my sister, my cousins, my friends. Moms had shown me that you just don't turn your back on your people. And when I looked at Fel with that silly, toothless grin, what could I do but claim her, love her?

There were days, though, when I just couldn't tolerate what my sister was doing to herself, and I had let her know it. One evening I was driving her and Moms home from a shopping trip when Fel kept nodding off to sleep. By then, she was gravely ill, but it was obvious to me that she was currently high. She'd slipped off to get her fix and didn't even care that our mother once again had to witness the aftereffects. I reached over to the passenger side, where Fel sat, and squeezed her hand, hard.

"I want you to wake up right now, or I'm kicking you the hell out of my car!" I demanded, as she struggled to crack her eyes. "You need to cut this shit out!"

After that, she disappeared for a few days, the way she often did when she knew she'd let her family down. Eventually, though, I quit fussing about the drugs and her lifestyle. I stopped trying to be the know-it-all doctor full of advice and warnings about what could happen if she didn't stop this or that. I tried to focus on just being baby bro, grateful for whatever time the two of us had left. This way, practically every time I saw her, she was her usual, cheery self. And this was the Fel I wanted to remember.

Beneath her smile, I knew she was really scared. She grew weaker with every bout of sickness, eventually not bouncing back as quickly. Sometimes, she would hug me as though she were trying to squeeze the life out of me, right into her own body.

"Marshall, I don't want to die," she'd say, holding me tighter than seemed possible for someone so frail. "I don't want to die!"

I hugged her back, wishing I could offer some assurance. But I braced myself for what I knew would soon come.

In fall 2001, Fellease developed an intestinal infection, which caused a bowel obstruction. Once again, she was admitted to Beth

Israel, where she had surgery to remove part of her intestine. She never fully recovered from that, and soon landed at St. Michael's Medical Center, one of three major hospitals in Newark.

One of their emergency room doctors buzzed me on my cell the afternoon of October 13. Fellease was critical, he said, and the family needed to get there right away. I was in my third year of residency and had made that call to families more times than I could count. I knew automatically what it meant: My big sister was either close to death or already gone. As a doctor, you don't want to deliver such devastating news over the phone, so you say just enough to get the family there. This time, I was on the other side.

Hang on, Fel, please, hang on. That's all I could think as I dashed the few miles from my place to my mother's house and then sped with her and my brother Carlton to the hospital. The ride was so quiet, it felt like all three of us were holding our breaths. When we arrived, I told the security guard in the emergency department waiting room that we'd received a call telling us to come. A nurse suddenly appeared to escort us to Fellease's room. She paused outside the door and broke the news: My sister had gone into cardiac arrest about an hour earlier, and the medical staff had been unable to revive her.

I took a deep breath, trying to prepare myself mentally to walk into that room.

"I'm sorry for your loss," the nurse said softly.

Even when you've said those words to others a million times, nothing can prepare you to hear them yourself. They made my knees weak. I hadn't had a chance to say good-bye. My heart ached as I took my mother's hand and moved quietly with her and Carlton to Fel's bedside. A breathing tube still hung limply from Fel's mouth, and her eyes were partially open. The doctor in me leaned over and gently pressed her eyelids shut. The little brother wept.

"Rest in peace," I whispered, wiping away my tears.

Tears streamed from Moms's eyes as she stroked Fel's thin hair. I could only imagine the magnitude of her grief. A parent isn't supposed to bury a child. No matter the circumstances, losing one must feel like losing part of your future. Carlton touched Fel's arm. I wrapped my fingers around her cold hand, and for a few moments, the three of us stood there silently, each with our private thoughts and tears.

Fel was just forty-two. I couldn't help thinking: *This didn't have to be. She didn't have to die this way.*

I tried to conjure up the sound of her voice and the sight of her smile before they were changed by AIDS. I thought about the many times she'd breathed life back into my hopes and dreams when I'd felt deflated, wanting so badly to quit during medical school. Now standing at her deathbed, I wanted to be a miracle worker and do the same for her, bring her back, healthy and whole. But all that anybody could do had been done.

Throughout her life, Fel had been my muse. In death, she is that once again. It is her face I see when I read the dreadful statistics. And it is her loss I feel when I tell young brothers and sisters: "Wrap your stuff up. Protect yourselves. One moment of passion isn't worth the risk of losing your life."

Common Sexually Transmitted Infections

The surest way to avoid transmission of STIs is to abstain from sexual contact or to be in a long-term, mutually monogamous relationship with a partner who has been tested and is known to be uninfected. Latex male condoms, when used consistently and correctly, can reduce the risk of transmission.

CHLAMYDIA

The most frequently reported bacterial sexually transmitted infection in the United States.

Symptoms: Usually absent or mild and may appear within one to three weeks after exposure; they include abnormal vaginal or penile discharge, burning sensation during urination, lower abdominal pain, low back pain, nausea, fever, painful intercourse, bleeding between menstrual periods, rectal pain, rectal discharge, or rectal bleeding.

Treatment: Antibiotics

GENITAL HERPES

A sexually transmitted infection caused by the herpes simplex viruses type 1 (HSV-1) or type 2 (HSV-2); HSV-2 causes most genital herpes.

Symptoms: Minimal or none, but can appear as one or more blisters on or around the genitals or rectum. The blisters break, leaving tender ulcers (sores) that may take two to four weeks to heal the first time they occur. May include a second crop of sores and flu-like symptoms, including fever and swollen glands.

Treatment: No cure, but antiviral medications can shorten and prevent outbreaks. Daily suppressive therapy for symptomatic herpes can reduce transmission to partners.

Health Concerns: First episode can produce several (typically four or five) outbreaks (symptomatic recurrences) within a year, but the recurrences usually decrease in frequency over time. Can cause recurrent painful genital sores in many adults, and herpes infection can be severe in people with suppressed immune systems. Frequently causes psychological distress in those who know they are infected. Can lead to potentially fatal infections in babies. In rare cases, the herpes virus can enter the brain and cause encephalitis, an extremely rare but serious brain disease.

GONORRHEA

A very common infection caused by a bacterium that can grow and multiply easily in the warm, moist areas of the reproductive tract.

Symptoms: No symptoms for most women and some men, but when they do appear: burning sensation during urination; penile discharge that is white, yellow, or green; swollen and painful testicles; increased vaginal discharge or vaginal bleeding between periods; rectal itching; rectal soreness; rectal bleeding; painful bowel movements; sore throat.

Treatment: Antibiotics

Health Concerns: If untreated in women, it may cause reproductive problems; in men, it can cause epididymitis, a painful condition of the ducts attached to the testicles that may lead to infertility. Can spread to the blood or joints, which can become life-threatening. Can be passed from an infected pregnant woman to her baby, where it can cause blindness, joint infection, or a life-threatening blood infection.

HIV/AIDS

HIV damages a person's body by destroying specific blood cells that are crucial to helping the body fight diseases. AIDS is the late stage of HIV infection, when a person's immune system is severely damaged and has difficulty fighting diseases, including certain cancers.

Symptoms: None, or flu-like symptoms within a few weeks of infection.

Treatment: Current combinations of medications can limit or slow down the destruction of the immune system and improve the health of people living with HIV, and may reduce their ability to transmit the virus. Most common HIV tests use blood to detect infection. Tests using saliva or urine are also available. Some tests take a few days for results, but there are also rapid HIV tests that can give results in about twenty minutes. Positive HIV tests must be followed up by a second test to confirm the positive result, a process that can take a few days to a few weeks.

Health Concerns: Early HIV infection is associated with many diseases, including cardiovascular disease, kidney disease, liver disease, and cancer.

HUMAN PAPILLOMAVIRUS (HPV)

The most common sexually transmitted infection.

Symptoms: None

Treatment: None for the virus itself, but there *are* treatments for the diseases that HPV can cause. Vaccines can protect males and females against some of the most common types of HPV that can lead to disease and cancer. The vaccines are given in three shots. For best protection, it's important to take all three doses. The vaccines are most effective when received at eleven or twelve years of age. Talk to a doctor about the appropriate one.

Health Concerns: In 90 percent of cases, the body's immune system clears HPV naturally within two years. If not cleared, can cause: genital warts, throat warts (respiratory papillomatosis), cervical cancer, or other less common cancers of the vulva, vagina, penis, anus, and oropharynx (back of throat, including base of tongue and tonsils).

PELVIC INFLAMMATORY DISEASE

Refers to infection of the uterus (womb), fallopian tubes (tubes that carry eggs from the ovaries to the uterus), and other reproductive organs.

Symptoms: Subtle or none; or lower abdominal pain, fever, bleeding, and pain in the right upper abdomen (rare).

Treatment: Antibiotics

Women who douche may have a higher risk of developing PID, compared with women who do not. Douching changes the vaginal flora (organisms that live in the vagina) in harmful ways, and can force bacteria from the vagina into the upper reproductive organs. Women who have an intrauterine device (IUD) may have a slightly increased risk of PID near the time of insertion, compared with women using other contraceptives or no contraceptive at all. Risk is greatly reduced if a woman is tested and, if necessary, treated for STIs before an IUD is inserted.

Health Concerns: Can damage the fallopian tubes and tissues in and near the uterus and ovaries and lead to serious consequences, including infertility, ectopic pregnancy (a pregnancy in the fallopian tube or elsewhere outside of the womb), abscess formation, and chronic pelvic pain.

SYPHILIS

Bacterial infection that is often called "the great imitator" because so many of its signs and symptoms are indistinguishable from those of other diseases.

Symptoms: Sores occur mainly on the external genitals, vagina, anus, or in the rectum. Sores also can occur on the lips and in the mouth. May present no symptoms for years, yet sufferers remain at risk for late complications if they are not treated. Also may include paralysis, numbness, gradual blindness, dementia, difficulty coordinating muscle movements, or death.

The primary stage is usually marked by the appearance of a single sore (called a "chancre"), but there may be multiple sores. The time between infection and the start of the first symptom can range from ten to ninety days (average twenty-one days).

Skin rash and mucous membrane lesions characterize the second-ary stage, which typically starts with the development of a rash on one or more areas of the body. The typical secondary syphilis rash appears as rough, red, or reddish brown spots both on the palms of the hands and the bottoms of the feet. But rashes with a different appearance may occur on other parts of the body. Other symptoms include fever, swollen lymph glands, sore throat, patchy hair loss, headaches, weight loss, muscle aches, and fatigue. The signs and symptoms of secondary syphilis will resolve with or without treat-ment, but without treatment the infection will progress to the latent (hidden) and possibly late stages of the disease.

Treatment: A single intramuscular injection of penicillin, an anti-biotic, if infection is less than a year. Additional doses are needed for someone who has had syphilis for longer than a year. For people who are allergic to penicillin, other antibiotics are available for treat-ment.

Health Concerns: In the late stages, the disease may subsequently damage the internal organs, including the brain, nerves, eyes, heart, blood vessels, liver, bones, and joints.

TRICHOMONIASIS (TRICH)
Common infection caused by a protozoan parasite.

Symptoms: None; itching or irritation inside the penis, burning after urination or ejaculation, discharge from penis; itching, burning, redness, or soreness of female genitals, discomfort with urination, thin discharge with unusual smell, uncomfortable sex.

Treatment: Laboratory test needed for diagnosis; can sometimes be cured with a single dose of prescription antibiotics.

Health Concerns: Preterm delivery in pregnant women.

FOR MORE INFORMATION:

Division of STD Prevention (DSTDP)

Centers for Disease Control and Prevention

www.cdc.gov/std

Order Publication Online at www.cdc.gov/std/pubs

CDC-INFO Contact Center

1-800-CDC-INFO (1-800-232-4636)

Email: cdcinfo@cdc.gov

Source: The Centers for Disease Control and Prevention's Division of STD Prevention

6

BABY LOVE

One unforgettable winter day in 2002, I knocked on the door of A3 and found a friendly couple waiting for me. The husband, a bank executive, was tall and well dressed. His wife, an elementary school teacher, didn't look anywhere near the age listed on her chart, thirty-nine. Classy and attractive, even in a hospital gown, she smiled and nodded as I introduced myself. Studying her chart, I could see that the patient, Mrs. Givens, was experiencing vaginal bleeding and abdominal cramps. I assumed she was pregnant, since the chart stated that her last menstrual period had been nine weeks earlier.

It didn't take long to discover that she was the more outspoken of the couple.

"Doctor, we are hardworking people," she began, sitting upright on the examining table. "We pay our tithes and rarely question God's reason for our failure to have a baby."

She was dry-eyed and calm.

"This is my sixth pregnancy, but I have no children," she continued. "There is nothing that I want more than to have a child. I've read books, attended seminars on parenting; I'm ready to be a mom."

But repeatedly she had miscarried. Her doctors could give her no explanation. That morning had started out fine, she said, but her heart sank when she got to work and discovered she was bleeding. She left work immediately and went home to lie down and pray. Unfortunately, though, soon she started feeling stomach cramps. She called her husband, who came home and rushed her to the hospital.

"Here, you should take a look at this," Mrs. Givens said, handing me a worn brown book—a journal, organized by dates, describing every detail of this and her previous pregnancies. She'd highlighted everything from her last menstrual period to prayer services. The journal provided an extraordinarily thorough look at her medical history. As I read some of the entries, Mr. Givens stood behind his wife like a bodyguard. The two of them seemed to have a close and loving relationship.

I noticed that Mrs. Givens had starred the date of a previous positive pregnancy test, and then I skipped to an entry six weeks later: "I prayed and prayed that it wouldn't happen," I read. "The bleeding started this morning. I rushed to the emergency department. This is our fourth time. I knew that I was miscarrying, but hoped maybe the doctors could save this one. I did everything I was told. I don't know if I can do this again."

I was still thumbing through the journal when Mrs. Givens interrupted. "Doctor, last time, the doctor told me they couldn't do anything. That was two years ago. My husband and I have been married for eight years. I can't lose another pregnancy. This is our last try. I said I would try until I'm forty, then no more."

She repeated it firmly: "After my fortieth birthday, no more tries."

I tried to sound optimistic. "Mrs. Givens, before making assumptions, let's finish your history and perform a physical exam. We'll order some lab work and perform an ultrasound to see where we are with this pregnancy."

"What was your name again?" she asked.

"Dr. Davis," I reminded her.

Mrs. Givens wasn't done with her story yet. "Dr. Davis, we have relatives and friends who are now on their second and third children. Every time I visit my cousins and friends, I wonder why—why can't we have the same joy?"

She had truly believed God would see her through, but I could see her faith starting to bend. "What's wrong with me? If only I could make it past the twenty-sixth week," she said.

Clearly she knew that at twenty-six weeks most premature babies have a decent chance at survival. But on this day, she was only seven weeks pregnant, eight at best.

"Today isn't happening," she said dully.

She quizzed me about whether she could have a "cervical cerclage," a medical procedure in which the cervix is practically sewn shut to keep it from opening prematurely and expelling the growing fetus. I could see that Mrs. Givens knew her stuff, had collected a ton of information. I explained that while the cerclage is a great option in some cases, she wasn't advanced enough in her pregnancy to consider it. A normal pregnancy lasts thirty-seven to forty-two weeks. Every week is a necessary phase in the development of an organ or body part, I said. Science has yet to discover a way to shorten the pregnancy process.

"At an early stage the body miscarries for many reasons, whether it's anatomical, your body structure, or something wrong with the fetus, like genetic abnormalities," I told her. "It's the body's way of handling such situations."

I sensed that she felt somehow to blame, and so I assured her she had not done anything wrong and that, in fact, from what I read in her journal, I could tell she'd been one of the most careful and deliberate pregnant women I'd seen. But Mrs. Givens seemed to be devolving right in front of me, suddenly becoming withdrawn, wrapping her arms around herself, and slowly rocking back and forth.

I glanced down at my watch and realized I had to move things along. Calling for a nurse to assist me, I wheeled my stool over so I could perform a pelvic exam. Once I placed the speculum, I could see a steady flow of maroon blood rushing out of Mrs. Givens's cervix. Not good. The bleeding likely meant she was shedding her uterine lining, fetus included. Probing with my hands, I could tell the cervix was closed. At least that was a good sign. An open cervix would have certainly signified an impending miscarriage. Perhaps bed rest could save the baby. A small chance, but a chance nonetheless.

Now I needed a more detailed look inside. I called for an orderly to take Mrs. Givens for an ultrasound. I could have performed the test myself but decided to spare her the indignity of possibly having to undergo the same test twice in one day: If she had indeed miscarried, hospital rules required her to have an ultrasound in the radiology suite. Since the Givenses would be busy for a while, I left to continue my rounds.

I picked up the chart for my next patient and knocked on A4's door, waited for a positive response, then stepped inside. A twenty-one-year-old woman, Ms. Harris, was pacing the small exam room. She was wearing a hospital gown, and I could easily see her behind, as she had failed to tie the gown in back. She was not happy; that much was plain.

"About time," she said, by way of introduction.

"Hi, I'm Dr. Davis," I said, pointing to my identification badge.

"I know who you are. I saw you running around the department last time I was here. I got a female doctor then. Is there one here today?"

I informed her that the female physician on staff would not be in until later. "At midnight—just another four hours, if you're willing to wait," I said, pretty sure what her response would be.

She made a hissing sound. "I guess you'll have to do. I was here a week ago. That doctor, she told me I was miscarrying."

I glanced down at the nurse's triage sheet and saw that the patient indeed was pregnant. An ultrasound performed a week earlier showed her at about seven weeks.

"She said I had a fifty-fifty chance of miscarrying," Ms. Harris continued. "That my ultrasound was abnormal, and then something about me having a threatened pregnancy. She told me to stay in bed and follow up with the clinic across the street from me."

"Well, have you made an appointment there?" I asked.

"No," she quipped. "I don't have time to show up at nobody's clinic."

She explained that she was too busy for a full doctor's appointment. "This is my sixth pregnancy," she said. She had three children at home and had undergone two abortions. "I only decided to come back today because I didn't miscarry. That doctor, she told me the baby would be gone by now."

She couldn't afford an abortion, she said, so she'd come back to the emergency room to get the procedure done. "After all, you guys told me it would happen, and it didn't," she added belligerently. "This is malpractice to me, and I want you to be the first to know that you guys lied to me and if I have to, I will get a lawyer."

I could barely believe her; I just hoped my facial expression didn't give away my thoughts. The memory of what had just happened next door was too fresh in my mind. It certainly affected my reaction to Ms. Harris—she was almost too much to take. My many encounters with young women like her sometimes left me feeling defeated, frustrated, as it seems impossible to stamp out all the reproductive ignorance and sexual carelessness in the world.

Looking back, I wish I'd taken a deep breath, ignored her rant, and talked to her about responsible methods of birth control to prevent unwanted pregnancies. I also wish I hadn't made any knee-jerk assumptions. I think we doctors sometimes assume too much.

We assume that young women know what to do for their bodies and are just behaving irresponsibly. Unfortunately, I'm too often reminded that, in fact, they *don't* have the information they need to make responsible choices, and that their sexual decisions are sometimes not just spontaneous but also based on myths and half-truths.

"Ms. Harris, I'm sorry to hear what happened, and I assure you we will find out what's going on," I said. "Now, to make sure I understand: You were hoping to lose this pregnancy and were under the impression that was going to happen."

"You got it," she said. "But since the bleeding stopped and I didn't see any clots, I'm sure it is still inside of me . . . Doc, I need this thing to happen, like, yesterday. I didn't want to come back here."

She continued: "You got to understand, I love my man, and he doesn't want any more kids." He already had six, she said, including her three, and they definitely didn't need any more mouths to feed.

I rubbed my suddenly tired eyes. "Ms. Harris, let's first see if you're still pregnant. You may have already miscarried, and the stopping of the vaginal bleeding may simply be a sign that the fetus has passed. I'll need to perform a full examination, which includes a pelvic. A nurse will be in the room with me."

"Oh, no, Dr. Davis, they did that exam last week. You don't have to repeat it. Besides, my man isn't going to allow no dude to look up inside of me."

As crazy as it sounds, this kind of response isn't rare. I've had patients demand to be examined only by a female doctor, and I've seen boyfriends and husbands act out, as though I was invading their personal Fort Knox. Usually, I can calm the situation by remaining professional, assuring the couple that I've performed thousands of pelvic exams and that a nurse (most assuredly a woman in these circumstances) would be present the entire time. Still, I'd seen grown men storm out of the room, slamming the door behind them.

"Ms. Harris, you're here for help. Let me do my job. The nurse will be in the room. You will be safe," I said more sharply than I'd intended.

"Okay, but if he comes in here and sees you doing this thing, he's going to get you," she threatened. I wanted to laugh out loud, even though it was obvious she was dead serious. Instead, I said calmly: "Let me worry about that, Ms. Harris."

I had her climb on the exam table and moved to listen to her lungs, which were clear. Her heart rate was regular, with no murmur. Her abdomen was soft, she had regular bowel sounds, there were no abnormal masses and no tenderness. "Okay, Ms. Harris, your exam thus far is fine. I'll go grab a nurse and be right back."

As I made my way to the door, she said, "Hey, Doctor, if you can't perform the abortion, do you have a department that'll do it for me? I really want to get it done today."

"Let's just get through the exam," I said, opening the door. "I'll also bring back the ultrasound machine."

As soon as I shut the door behind me, I couldn't contain my disbelief. Linda, one of my favorite nurses, was standing near the door. Her expression told me she could tell something was wrong.

"I'm going to need you as a chaperone in A4," I explained. "You won't believe what's going on in there. I've got an irate patient blaming us because she *didn't* miscarry."

Rolling the ultrasound machine toward the room, I explained the two stories unfolding simultaneously. "What's crazy is that the couple in A3 would kill for the opportunity to have a baby, and here we have Ms. Harris, who can't wait to abort her fetus."

I wasn't judging either family, I told Linda. Ms. Harris had every right to get an abortion, just not in the emergency room. I wished these young couples thought more about birth control before it came to this. And I wished I had the power to grant both parties their desires: If only I could take Ms. Harris's unwanted pregnancy and give it to Mr. and Mrs. Givens.

"That would be a miracle," Linda said.

Well, it was definitely pure fantasy. And this here was as real as life got. I completed Ms. Harris's ultrasound, which showed that she was indeed still pregnant. There was even fetal heart activity.

"Ms. Harris, the fetus is still present. As you can see from the image on the ultrasound machine, the heart is beating."

"I don't want to see it. I want it out of me."

"Ms. Harris, we don't perform abortions in the emergency department. You'll have to follow up with the obstetrics clinic."

There wasn't much left for me to say to her, although silently a million thoughts were spinning in my mind. I usually wouldn't have gotten so worked up, but the side-by-side contrast was just so stark. Though I was taken aback by Ms. Harris's irritation, part of me understood. To her, this fetus represented one thing: more struggle in a young life already heaped with so much of it. I got it. I really did. I just wanted her to see the other side, and before I could bite it back, a non-medical opinion slipped out of my mouth: "You know, there are people out there who wish they were in your position."

"What do you mean?" she snapped.

I chose my words carefully. "Well, some women can't have kids and want more than anything else to be a mom."

Immediately, I wished I'd kept my mouth shut. She looked shocked at first, and then her face contorted to anger: "Dr. Davis, you have some nerve. You are not the judge of me. It's none of your business what I decide to do."

I apologized right away. I hadn't intended to offend her. I'm not sure she heard me, though, because by then her voice had reached a full screech: "I'm going to sue this hospital! I hope it burns to the ground!"

I left the room, stood outside for a moment, and took a deep breath. The Givenses were waiting to hear the results of the ultrasound, so I retrieved their chart and headed back to A3. The hour it had taken for me to get the ultrasound results had given the couple some good time together, apparently. Mrs. Givens seemed more at peace. Her husband sat on the bed beside her and held her hand. I felt like a judge about to render a disappointing verdict. My words would redefine their lives somehow and determine the road they would take from here.

Sweat began beading on my forehead. I had removed my white coat earlier so that I would look less formal, less callous. I only hoped my scrubs didn't smell, since I hadn't had time to wash them the night before.

"Mr. and Mrs. Givens, the ultrasound results show a low-lying fetus close to the cervix," I began.

"What does that mean?" Mrs. Givens asked.

I knew beforehand that they wouldn't understand the medical terminology. I guess I was just trying to buy more time. I didn't want to steal their dreams. This part of my job sucked.

"Mrs. Givens, you are miscarrying. The fetus is moving toward the vagina, and eventually you will pass it."

The husband and wife reached for each other, crying. For me, it was bad enough being the bearer of bad news, but I especially hated that this couple's strong faith had not been rewarded—at least, not yet. I searched my brain for comforting words.

"I read your journal," I told them. "The two of you are believers and an inspiration to me. Please don't blame yourselves. All the right steps were taken. Your journal tells it all, from your battle with morning sickness to the fact that Mr. Givens slept in the guest room when he had the flu so that you wouldn't get sick. So many sacrifices. You are going to be great parents, even if you have to adopt."

I had no idea whether Mr. and Mrs. Givens had ever even considered adoption or would in the future, but I hoped so. I'd seen far too many children come into the world unwanted, and—as far as I could see—this husband and wife were a loving couple who wanted nothing more than to become parents.

For many couples, the desire for a blood connection to a child, to create someone who carries part of their unique genetic makeup, is so strong that they don't even want to hear about adoption. Many are afraid. They wonder: *Can I love a child who has no biological part of me? How will I know for sure what the child is like? What if I end up with a problem child?* Those fears are real, and unfortunately a few highly visible stories about adoptions gone wrong contribute to broad misperceptions. But adoption, much like having a child the natural way, is full of wonder and mystery. There is no 100 percent guarantee that a family who adopts will wind up with a perfect child and a perfect life, just as there is no guarantee that a natural birth will result in these things. But the 2007 National Survey of Adoptive Parents, the first large national survey of families across all adoption types—the foster care system, private domestic adoptions, and international adoptions—offers some assurance.

Conducted by the U.S. Department of Health and Human Services, the study—which included interviews with more than 2,000 families—shows that the overwhelming majority of adoptive families are happy with their choice: 93 percent of those who adopted through private agencies reported that they would definitely make the same decision again; 87 percent of those who had adopted internationally also said they would do so again; and 81 percent of those who had gone through the foster care system would repeat their decision as well.

Likewise, a large majority—85 percent—of the adopted children were reported by their parents to have been in excellent or very good health. Eighty-eight percent of the school-aged children demonstrated positive social behaviors. Only a small minority had been diagnosed with disorders such as attachment disorder, depression, attention deficit disorder, attention deficit/hyperactivity disorder, conduct disorder, Fetal Alcohol Syndrome, or drug issues. That's the happy side of the adoption coin, the side that the public rarely sees.

The need for more African American families to adopt is tremendous, given the disproportionate numbers of our children in the nation's foster care system waiting to find a permanent family. As of the end of September 2010, there were a total of 107,011 children in foster care available for adoption—30,812 of whom were African American and another 6,771 of mixed race.

The process for becoming an adoptive parent varies, depending on the type of adoption. But all adoptions generally require some type of home study, in which an investigator, usually a social worker, conducts a series of home visits and interviews with family members and collects pertinent data to determine a family's fitness to become adoptive parents. Of the three adoption types, the foster care system is the most affordable, with fees that generally don't exceed $2,500. A private adoption can cost upward from $5,000 to $40,000, and an international adoption from $15,000 to $30,000. The push in recent decades to increase the number of African American adoptive families has spawned an industry of agencies and programs dedicated to that purpose. Since faith plays such an important role in the lives of many black families, one of the most visible programs is connected to the Catholic Church. One Church One Child dates back to the 1980s, when Father George Clements, a civil rights activist and African American Roman Catholic priest, adopted a boy and formed the organization to encourage churches to help find stable homes for black children. Dozens of state and local chapters of the organization have since been formed throughout the country. For families of faith, like Mr. and Mrs. Givens, the support of their church in adopting a child would add an extra layer of comfort.

I've always heard that God works in mysterious ways. I couldn't give Mr. and Mrs. Givens the news they wanted in the emergency room that day. But maybe my role was broader: to plant the seed of possibility.

Birth Control Methods

CONTINUOUS ABSTINENCE

This means not having sex (vaginal, anal, or oral) *at any time*. It is the only sure way to prevent pregnancy and protect against sexually transmitted infections (STIs), including HIV.

NATURAL FAMILY PLANNING/RHYTHM METHOD

This method means either you do not have sex or you use a barrier method on the days you are most fertile (most likely to become pregnant). It also involves checking your cervical mucus and recording your body temperature each day. Cervical mucus is the discharge from your vagina. You are most fertile when it is clear and slippery like raw egg whites. Use a basal thermometer to take your temperature and record it on a chart: Your temperature will rise 0.4 to 0.8°F on the first day of ovulation. You can talk with your doctor or a natural family planning instructor to learn how to record and understand this information.

BARRIER METHODS—PUT UP A BLOCK, OR BARRIER, TO KEEP SPERM FROM REACHING THE EGG

Contraceptive sponge

This barrier method is a soft, disk-shaped device with a loop for removal. It is made out of polyurethane foam and contains nonoxynol-9, which kills sperm (spermicide). Before having sex, wet the sponge and place it, loop side down, inside your vagina to cover the cervix. The sponge is effective for up to twenty-four hours, including more than one act of intercourse. It needs to be left in for at least six hours after having sex to prevent pregnancy. It must then be taken out within thirty hours after it is inserted.

Only one kind of contraceptive sponge is sold in the United States: the Today Sponge. Women who are sensitive to the spermicide nonoxynol-9 should not use the sponge.

Diaphragm, cervical cap, and cervical shield

These barrier methods block the sperm from entering the cervix (the opening to your womb) and reaching the egg. Before having sex, add spermicide (to block or kill sperm) to the device. (You can buy spermicide gel or foam at a drugstore.) Then place it inside your vagina to cover your cervix. All three of these barrier methods must be left in place for six to eight hours after having sex to prevent pregnancy. The diaphragm should be taken out within twenty-four hours. The cap and shield should be taken out within forty-eight hours.

Female condom

This condom is worn by the woman inside her vagina. It keeps sperm from getting into her body. It is made of thin, flexible, man-made rubber and is packaged with a lubricant. It can be inserted up to eight hours before having sex. Use a new condom each time you have intercourse. And don't use it and a male condom at the same time. Condoms, both male and female, are the only methods listed here that also offer protection from STIs.

Male condom

A male condom is a thin sheath placed over an erect penis to keep sperm from entering a woman's body. Condoms can be made of latex, polyurethane, or "natural lambskin." The natural kind do not protect against STIs. Condoms work best when used with a vaginal spermicide, which kills the sperm. You need to use a new condom with each sex act.

HORMONAL METHODS—PREVENT PREGNANCY BY INTERFERING WITH OVULATION, FERTILIZATION, AND/OR IMPLANTATION OF THE FERTILIZED EGG

Oral contraceptives—combined pill ("the pill")

The pill contains the hormones estrogen and progestin. It is taken daily to keep the ovaries from releasing an egg. The pill also causes changes in the lining of the uterus and the cervical mucus to keep the sperm from joining the egg.

Many types of oral contraceptives are available. Talk with your doctor about which is best for you.

The patch

Also called by its brand name, Ortho Evra, this skin patch is worn on the lower abdomen, buttocks, outer arm, or upper body. It releases the hormones progestin and estrogen into the bloodstream to stop the ovaries from releasing eggs in most women. It also thickens the cervical mucus, which keeps the sperm from joining with the egg. You put on a new patch once a week for three weeks. The fourth week you don't use a patch in order to have a period.

Shot/injection

The birth control shot often is called by its brand name, Depo-Provera. With this method you get injections, or shots, of the hormone progestin in the buttocks or arm every three months. A new type is injected under the skin. The birth control shot stops the ovaries from releasing an egg in most women. It also causes changes in the cervix that keep the sperm from joining with the egg. The shot should not be used more than two years in a row because it can cause a temporary loss of bone density.

Vaginal ring

This is a thin, flexible ring that releases the hormones progestin and estrogen. It works by stopping the ovaries from releasing eggs. It also thickens the cervical mucus, which keeps the sperm from joining the egg. It is commonly referred to by its brand name, NuvaRing. You squeeze the ring between your thumb and index finger and insert it into your vagina. You wear the ring for three weeks, take it out for the week that you have your period, and then put in a new ring.

IMPLANTABLE DEVICES—DEVICES THAT ARE INSERTED INTO THE BODY AND LEFT IN PLACE FOR A FEW YEARS

Implantable rod

This is a matchstick-sized, flexible rod that is put under the skin of the upper arm. It is often called by its brand name, Implanon. The rod releases progestin, which causes changes in the lining of the uterus and the cervical mucus to keep the sperm from joining an egg. Less often, it stops the ovaries from releasing eggs. It is effective for up to three years.

Intrauterine devices or IUDs

An IUD is a small device shaped like a T that goes in your uterus. There are two types:

- **Copper IUD**—The copper IUD goes by the brand name ParaGard. It releases a small amount of copper into the uterus, which prevents the sperm from reaching and fertilizing the egg. If fertilization does occur, the IUD keeps the fertilized egg from implanting in the lining of the uterus. A doctor needs to put in your copper IUD. It can stay in your uterus for five to ten years.
- **Hormonal IUD**—The hormonal IUD goes by the brand name Mirena. It is sometimes called an "intrauterine system," or IUS. It releases progestin into the uterus, which keeps the ovaries from releasing an egg and causes the cervical mucus to thicken so sperm can't

reach the egg. It also affects the ability of a fertilized egg to successfully implant in the uterus. A doctor needs to put in a hormonal IUD. It can stay in your uterus for up to five years.

PERMANENT BIRTH CONTROL METHODS—FOR PEOPLE WHO ARE SURE THEY NEVER WANT TO HAVE A CHILD OR DO NOT WANT MORE CHILDREN

Sterilization implant (Essure)

Essure is the first non-surgical method of sterilizing women. A thin tube is used to thread a tiny spring-like device through the vagina and uterus into each fallopian tube. The device works by causing scar tissue to form around the coil. This blocks the fallopian tubes and stops the egg and sperm from joining. It can take about three months for the scar tissue to grow, so it's important to use another form of birth control during this time. Then you will have to return to your doctor for a test to see if scar tissue has fully blocked your tubes.

Surgical sterilization

For women, surgical sterilization closes the fallopian tubes by cutting, tying, or sealing them. This stops the eggs from going down to the uterus where they can be fertilized. The surgery can be done a number of ways. Sometimes, a woman having cesarean birth has the procedure done at the same time, so as to avoid having additional surgery later.

For men, having a vasectomy keeps sperm from going to his penis, so his ejaculate never has any sperm in it. Sperm stays in the system after surgery for about three months. During that time, use a backup form of birth control to prevent pregnancy. A simple test can be done to check if all the sperm is gone; it is called a "semen analysis."

EMERGENCY CONTRACEPTION—USED IF A WOMAN'S PRIMARY METHOD OF BIRTH CONTROL FAILS. IT SHOULD *NOT* BE USED AS A REGULAR METHOD OF BIRTH CONTROL.

Plan B One-Step or Next Choice. It is also called "the morning after pill."

Emergency contraception keeps a woman from getting pregnant when she has had unprotected vaginal intercourse. Emergency contraception can be taken as a single pill treatment or in two doses. A single dose treatment works as well as two doses and does not have more side effects. It works by stopping the ovaries from releasing an egg or keeping the sperm from joining with the egg. For the best chances for it to work, take the pill as soon as possible after unprotected sex. It should be taken within seventy-two hours after having unprotected sex. A single-pill dose or two-pill dose of emergency contraception is available over-the-counter (OTC) for women ages seventeen and older.

All birth control methods work best if used correctly and every time you have sex. Be sure you know the right way to use them. Sometimes doctors don't explain how to use a method because they assume you already know. Talk with your doctor if you have questions. They are used to talking about birth control. For more information about birth control methods, call womenshealth.gov at 800-994-9662 (TDD: 888-220-5446) or contact the following organizations:

- **American College of Obstetricians and Gynecologists**
  Phone: 800-762-2264 x 349 (for publications requests only)
- **Food and Drug Administration**
  Phone: 888-463-6332
- **Planned Parenthood Federation of America**
  Phone: 800-230-7526
- **Population Council**
  Phone: 212-339-0500

Source: All of the birth control information in the preceding pages was reprinted from womenshealth.gov, a federal government website managed by the U.S. Department of Health and Human Services Office on Women's Health.

Adoption Types

There are four basic types of adoption:

- public agency adoption
- domestic private agency adoption
- international adoption
- independent adoption

As the chart below shows, requirements, costs, and timing vary between and within the different types of adoption. To decide which is best for you, think seriously about the type of child you would like to adopt (for example, an infant, an older child or group of siblings, a child from another country, a child who has special needs, etc.).

Type of Adoption	Definition	Children Available	Approximate Cost	Who Can Adopt	How Long It Takes
Public agency adoption	an adoption directed and supervised by a state or local Department of Human Services (or Social Services, or Human Resources, or Health and Welfare, or Child and Family Services, etc.)	children with special needs (kids who are harder to place due to emotional or physical disorders, age, race, member- ship in a sibling group, backgrounds); rarely infants	from $0 to $2,500 (depending on the state, up to $2,000 of "non- recurring" adoption costs for eligible special needs children may be reimbursed)	flexible eligibility re- quirements for adoptive parents; on a case-by- case basis, will consider single parents, parents over the age of forty, parents who have other children, parents with low incomes, etc.	starts slowly, but for those who have an updated home study, placement can occur as soon as a few months after selecting a child
Private agency adoption	an adoption directed and supervised by a privately funded, licensed adoption agency	sometimes handle special needs chil- dren; more commonly associated with younger children and infants	$5,000 to $40,000; lower for special needs children; some agencies have sliding fee scales	agencies may recruit parents based on race, religious affiliation, etc.; for infant adoptions, birth mother often chooses	a few months to a few years (sometimes longer for in- fant adoption)

Type of Adoption	Definition	Children Available	Approximate Cost	Who Can Adopt	How Long It Takes
International adoption (not legal in all states; also known as "private adoption")	process of adopting a child who is not a U.S. citizen, which may be accomplished privately through an attorney or through an international adoption agency	nearly seventy countries allow their children to be adopted by U.S. citizens; ages range from infants to teens; health conditions vary	$15,000 to $30,000 (varies by country; travel and travel-related expenses may be additional)	depends on agency and country requirements; some countries will accept single parents; most prospective parents are between ages twenty-five and forty-five	six months to several years depending on the child's age and health and the country's political climate
Independent adoption	an adoption initiated by prospective parents and completed with help from an attorney or adoption counselor	generally infants	$8,000 to $40,000+ (includes prospective parents' cost of finding a birth mother, certain birth mother expenses, and attorney's fees)	birth mothers typically choose the adoptive parent—preferences tend to run toward younger, affluent, married couples	varies; as long as it takes to find a birth mother who will see the process through to finalization

* **Note:** It is also possible to adopt children by first becoming a foster parent; many children who have special needs are adopted by their foster parents. **Drawback:** There is no guarantee that foster parents will be able to adopt either the child in their care or any other child. Most children in foster care return to their birth families, and some are placed in the custody of relatives or adopted by parents the agency feels are best able to meet the child's particular needs. **Advantages:** Children who enter foster care are, on average, younger than children who become legally free for adoption after spending years in care. In addition, parents who take in foster children have time to get fully acquainted with a child before committing to adoption. The more parents know about a child, the better their chances are for a successful adoption.

Source: North American Council on Adoptable Children, 970 Raymond Ave., Suite 106, St. Paul, MN 55114, 651-644-3036, www.nacac.org. For a more comprehensive list of adoption agencies, go to: www.childwelfare.gov/nfcad/.

Agencies Specializing in African American Adoptions

African American Adoption Agency
2356 University Ave. W
St. Paul, MN 55114-1850
888-840-4084 or
651-659-0460
afadopt@afadopt.org
www.afadopt.org

African American Adoptions, Inc.
8471 Canyon Oak Drive
Springfield, VA 22153
703-829-5641
www.aaadoptions.org

Another Choice for Black Children, Inc.
2340 Beatties Ford Road
Charlotte, NC 28216
800-774-3534 or
704-394-1124
info@acfbc.org
www.acfbc.org

Ardythe and Gale Sayers Center for African American Adoption
2049 Ridge Ave.
Evanston, IL 60201
847-733-3209
www.cradle.org/
adoption-agency/
adopt_aa.html

The Black Adoption Placement and Research Center
2332 Merced St.
San Leandro, CA 94577
510-430-3600
family@baprc.org
www.baprc.org

Black Adoption Services Three Rivers Adoption Council
307 Fourth Ave., Ste. 310
Pittsburgh, PA 15222
412-471-8722
www.3riversadopt.org

Children's Bureau, Inc.
615 N. Alabama St.
Indianapolis, IN 46204
317-264-2700
www.childrensbureau
.org

Dallas Minority Adoption Council
P.O. Box 764058
Dallas, TX 75376-4058
214-371-5280
rosepo@baylorhealth
.edu

Dunbar Association, Inc.
1453 S. State St.
Syracuse, NY 13205
315-476-4269
www.dunbarassociation
.org/

Families First
1105 W. Peachtree St.,
NE
P.O. Box 7948, Stn. C
Atlanta, GA 30357-0948
404-853-2800
www.familiesfirst.org

Family Matters of Greater Washington, D.C.
1509 16th St. NW
Washington, DC 20036
202 289-1510
http://familymattersdc
.org/

Harlem Dowling-West Side Center
2090 Adam Clayton Powell Jr. Blvd.
New York, NY 10027
212-749-3656
www.harlemdowling.org

Homes for Black Children
511 E. Larned St.
Detroit, MI 48226
313-961-4777
www.homes4black
children.org

Institute for Black Parenting
1299 E. Artesia Blvd.
Carson, CA 90746
877-367-8858 or
   310-900-0930
www.blackparenting
   .org/services.html

Institute for Family & Child Well-Being
P.O. Box 7845
Upper Marlboro, MD
   20792
info@familyandchild
   wellbeing.com
www.familyandchild
   wellbeing.com

Minority Adoption Program Child Saving Institute
4545 Dodge St.
Omaha, NE 68132
402-553-6000 or
   866-400-4274
csiinfo@childsaving.org
www.childsaving.org

Mississippi Families for Kids
407 Briarwood Drive,
   Ste. 209
Jackson, MS 39206
601-957-7670
www.mffk.org

National Network of Adoption Advocacy Programs (NNAAP)
5601 Chamberlayne
   Road
Richmond, VA 23227
804-377-1627

The New York Chapter Association of Black Social Workers' Child Adoption Counseling and Referral Service
1969 Madison Ave.
New York, NY 10035
212-831-5181
abswnyc@aol.com

New York Council on Adoptable Children
589 Eighth Ave., 15th Fl.
New York, NY 10018
212-475-0222
www.coac.org

One Church One Child of North/North Central Texas
2860 Evans Ave.
Fort Worth, TX 76104
866-42-ADOPT
   (866-422-3678)
ococdfw@aol.com

Rejoice! Inc.
1820 Linglestown Rd.
Harrisburg, PA 17110
717-221-0722
www.rejoice-inc.org

Tabor Children's Services
57 E. Armat St.
Philadelphia, PA 19144
215-842-4800
www.tabor.org

Women's Christian Alliance
1722 Cecil B. Moore
   Ave.
Philadelphia, PA
   19121-3405
215-236-9911
www.wcafamily.org

7

CLUBBING

Beep. Beep. Beep. . . . I'd just about drifted off to sleep one night in late spring 2001 when the sound of my pager startled me. Instinctively, I jumped off the cot in the resident call room, the tiny quarters where young doctors can rest, and slid into my sneakers. I glanced down at the small electronic screen to find out what awaited me two flights down: a combative twenty-three-year-old male, gunshot wound to the abdomen, arriving in five minutes.

No time to stop at the sink or run through the shower to freshen up. Within seconds, I was standing at the elevator, pressing the button in rapid succession. It gave me something to do as I waited. When the door swung open, I jumped on board, rode to the ground floor, and ran toward the emergency department. Once there, I quickly put on a disposable yellow gown to cover my scrubs. This case would be bloody for sure, and I couldn't ruin the only pair of scrubs I had with me. I made it to the ambulance bay with the rest of the trauma team to await our patient. This was my second rotation at University Hospital's trauma center, and I was one of two visiting residents. The rest of the team included the chief trauma resident, the junior resident, and a couple of medical students.

Ron, the trauma nurse, was there, too. With two decades of

experience, he was the true leader of the department and got a kick out of us bambinos learning the field. Like many of the nurses, he would make biting remarks to prove that the nurses were the true kings and queens of this jungle. You couldn't show fear or weakness, or they would eat you alive. I'm sure they sat around most days laughing at the first-year residents (also called "interns"), wandering around the E.R., barely able to distinguish a stethoscope from a blood pressure cuff. An outsider could probably figure out our seniority just by our facial expressions and body language. The more confused and bewildered, the less experienced they were. The chief resident looked more exhausted than anything else, and the king of the jungle was looking for his prey. Ron's shift had just begun, which meant he was fresh and ready to torment one of the residents or medical students.

In an instant, the doors flung open, and the emergency medical technicians were rushing a stretcher toward us. The team quickly lifted our patient onto the gurney, and I used a huge pair of shears to cut off his clothes. Ron swooped in and barked at the intern: "Now, you know you don't know what you are doing, MOVE!" Within seconds, he had hooked the patient to a monitor, established a second IV, drawn blood for the lab, and placed a Foley catheter, while the rest of us assessed the damage.

Our patient, a young brother, was alive, but barely. The monitor picked up a heart rhythm, and as I placed my gloved hand into his groin region to find the femoral artery, I could feel a faint pulse. I inserted a large bore IV right next to the artery into the femoral vein, allowing us to pump in saline and blood. Blood gushed from the wounds in his chest and abdomen, toward his crotch, and my gloved hand was suddenly bright red. The junior resident moved in with a Number 11 scalpel to insert a chest tube, and the rest of the team completed our mental checklist, examining the patient for further injury. I counted three gunshot wounds, two to the abdomen and one to the chest. The X-ray technician moved in, giving us a quick look at things on the inside. The bullet appeared to have struck the spine, knocking its alignment off track, indicating a high probability of paralysis. The patient was rushed to the operating room. Finally, Ron retreated. As the stretcher disappeared around the corner toward the elevator, the intern fought back tears. Just one year removed from such status, I knew how overwhelmed she must have felt.

Moments later, I heard yelling on the other side of the department. Another young man was stumbling in, his white T-shirt drenched with blood—another shooting. He was a big guy, six feet two inches tall, roughly 250 pounds. A female companion was struggling to keep him upright; his legs were wobbling underneath his large frame. Then his feet gave way and he collapsed in the middle of the department. Ron quickly grabbed a stretcher. Newly regloved, the rest of the team rushed to the patient's side and tossed his limp body onto it. Ron whipped out a needle from his back pocket and established almost immediate IV access. Fluids were attached to the catheter and squeezed in. Ron was back on his throne, and his target, this go-around, was the junior resident.

"What the hell are you doing?" Ron yelled. "Get this guy intubated. Come on, let's go!"

Ron was as good as any trauma surgeon. In a pinch, he might have even been able to perform surgery—at least that's the kind of confidence he exuded. "Listen, if you can't do it, then move and let someone else."

Sweat formed on the junior resident's forehead as he pushed the tube into the patient's trachea. I checked for sounds of breathing and gave a thumbs-up, signaling that the tube was in the proper place. I believe the poor resident feared Ron more than missing the intubation. The medical student took my shears and removed the patient's jeans and bloody T-shirt. I inspected his body and found one gunshot wound in his abdomen. There were no bowel sounds, and his stomach was swollen to the size of a full-term pregnancy. He was surely bleeding inside. The chief resident placed a central line catheter into his neck. Ron hooked him up to the monitor, and we rolled him over for the standard back and rectal exam. The white sheet covering the black foam mattress was now a bright maroon. The patient's blood pressure was low, and his heart rate was fast. He was barely hanging on. I could see the attending trauma surgeon making his way through the department, and, like the parting of the Red Sea, everyone moved. This was the only time I saw Ron back down. It wasn't as much a retreat as a show of respect for a fellow king of the jungle. If challenged, though, Ron would rise up, and he and Dr. Langston would battle, right there in front of everyone. Dr. Langston looked at the chief resident and quickly uttered two words: "Let's go."

Eight more traumas came in that night—a total of twenty during my thirty-hour shift, not reaching my personal record of thirty-five. I was so drained that I welcomed the morning report, when all of the trauma docs, radiologists, nurses, and other staff gathered in a room to sign out the cases from the night before and hand over operations to the next team. This was the attending trauma surgeon's stage, as he drilled us, pointing out every mistake. The chief resident usually got it the worst, but no one was exempt. It was like a fraternity den, and hazing was allowed.

"You radiologists are fancy art critics," Dr. Langston joked while making his assessment of our performance the night before. "All you do is read pictures and offer your impressions."

I sat back in my seat, coffee in hand. Medical school had introduced me to the world of coffee, and I'd since become somewhat of a connoisseur. Even with the caffeine, I was struggling to keep my eyes open. The initials of all the patients from the night before were marked on the green board. The gunshot victim who had walked in with his female companion had made it out of the operating room—critical but alive. He needed more surgery. "Severe internal damage occurred, and he was unable to be closed up," the chief resident said. A plastic covering from a saline bag had been placed over his exposed abdomen to prevent bacteria from entering the body cavity.

Five patients, highlighted on the board by their initials, had one final update: DECEASED. My patient who'd come in with the three gunshot wounds was still alive but quite truculent. When he woke up from the anesthesia, he started yelling profanities, asking the nurses about the shooter and saying what he would do if the police didn't capture him. He was Mr. Tough Guy, a common attitude around Newark blocks that seemed to require that those who live there have an edge to survive. No sign of weakness was allowed. Healthwise, though, he appeared better off than the one who'd been shot just once. The number of times a person has been shot is always less important than the trajectory of the bullet.

It was about noon when we closed out the morning report and handed over the next thirty hours to the Trauma B team. I would report back to the hospital at 7:00 A.M. the following day with my team, Trauma A.

The sunshine outside was bright. It was going to be another warm day. I headed for my Honda Accord. That car was tough. Despite a few fender benders and even a couple of burglaries, she was still holding up, still reliable. She'd been broken in to so many times, I sometimes felt like I was borrowing her from the thieves. I'd mistakenly left the steering wheel lock off the last time she'd been stolen. The perpetrator was found two weeks later, asleep in the front seat. When the police finally contacted me, and I went to claim my car, it appeared the thief had been living inside. Empty French fry cartons, burger wrappings, liquor bottles, and drug paraphernalia littered the floor and seats. The guy behind the counter at the car lot told me I'd have to pay $210 to take her home. When I asked about the damage, he responded: "You pay here first and then you can see for yourself. You can sign the car over to us if you don't want to take it." He then pointed the dirty fingernail of his stubby index finger toward a sign that said: "NO Exceptions, Money First, Then Your Car."

The Honda was worth it. She had traveled with me from medical school to Newark, never giving up. Through it all, she had required only minimal repairs. I liked to think that the scratches, dents, and off-track front window added character to her ten-year-old body. I'd nicknamed her The Coupe. She'd gotten me not only to work, but in and out of New York regularly, never breaking down—as I feared she might—in the Holland Tunnel. Many times I'd entered the tunnel in New Jersey, fingers crossed, hoping to make it to the other side. I didn't want to be the guy that everybody who travels that route has seen—the one with the stalled old car paralyzing traffic in the tunnel, inciting furious horns and looks that could kill. The Coupe reminded me of me. We'd both been beaten up pretty badly, but we kept on pushing.

She was waiting for me in the parking lot after the morning report. As I drove home, I couldn't wait to get into bed. I lived less than fifteen minutes from the hospital, in a working-class neighborhood, where I rented a room in a three-story home owned by Carole Jackson. Her daughter, Mary Ann, who had been friends with George, Rameck, and me in high school, lived in a first-floor apartment connected to the house. Mary Ann had stayed in touch with George throughout college and dental school, and he'd told her that I was moving back to Newark for my residency and was looking for an affordable place to stay. She'd asked her mother if she'd be willing to rent me the vacant third-floor bedroom. The setup was perfect. I had no savings and no intention of moving back home with my mother, which would have meant sharing a room with my younger brother. A place of my own would symbolize my fresh start, and a room was about all I could afford.

When we'd been in high school, Mrs. Jackson had been the active PTA mom that all the kids knew and loved. She remembered me and welcomed me into her home. She was like my mom in that way: She always had a house full of relatives and friends, some of whom stayed with her from time to time and others who just popped in occasionally for one of her delicious home-cooked meals. That, of course, made me feel right at home. My room was nothing fancy, but just right for me: a double bed, a dresser, and a desk. There was also a window, which I covered with black curtains to block the sunlight on days like this, when my shift ended in the middle of the day and I needed to hibernate until it was time to rise and do it all again.

That day, I headed straight to my room and slept for six straight hours. When the aroma from the kitchen told me it was dinnertime, I stumbled down to the kitchen. Mrs. Jackson was standing there, smiling.

"I was just about to tell Frankie to wake you," she said, referring to her middle-aged niece, who lived in another room on the third floor. "Another long night, huh?"

"Yeah, they kept coming, all night long," I said.

She pointed to a pan of freshly grilled salmon on the stove. "Well, have some of this," she said. "I brought it today from the market."

I inhaled my meal of fish, mashed potatoes, and string beans, then retired back to my dungeon and slept through the night. At 6:00 A.M. Sunday, my alarm blared. I dragged myself out of my squeaky bed and headed to the bathroom down the hall. The forty-five-watt lightbulb gave the hallway a tunnel-like feel, and the pipes growled in the bathroom as I turned on the hot water. I showered quickly, changed into a new pair of scrubs, and threw an extra pair in my bag so I wouldn't get caught off guard again with back-to-back bloody traumas and no change of clothes.

I had to hurry if I wanted a cup of coffee before the morning report. I rushed to the cafeteria, and the first person I saw was Ron. We greeted each other cheerfully. Ron liked me, I think because we were both from Newark and shared both love and concern for our city. He talked to me often about his son and how proud he was of him. I'm sure it must have bothered him, too, to see so many young men who looked like us passing through the E.R.

I glanced up and saw the chief resident at the oatmeal stand. She still looked exhausted. I wondered if she had been able to rest on her day off. She was in her last year of residency, married, with a son and daughter. I couldn't imagine raising a family during this time. She and I met up at the cash register.

"Good morning, young doctors," said Mrs. Wallace, the cashier and matriarch at University. She'd been working there for thirty-five years. Even the senior docs greeted her with warmth. She was one of the few constants at the hospital, having known many of the doctors now inching toward retirement since they were residents. We made our way to morning report. The room was crowded; some staffers were standing, as there were never enough seats. The senior doctors occupied the front of the room; the chief resident from Trauma B stood at the podium. He was shifting nervously from side to side. Glancing up at the board, I noted twenty more trauma cases from the night before, and seven deaths. The two patients I'd treated in my previous shift were still alive. The condition of the first one, the guy brought in by ambulance with multiple gunshot wounds, had been upgraded, and he was now in a regular room, out of the Surgical Intensive Care Unit. The second one, who'd walked in with the young woman, had taken a turn for the worse, though. He was scheduled for additional surgery later in the day to remove more of his intestines.

The chief resident filled us in on what he'd learned about our gunshot patients from the police, who had been notified by the hospital as usual after a shooting. I initially suspected that there had been a gun battle between Patient One and Patient Two, but I couldn't have been more wrong. The two were actually brothers who had been out at a local nightclub. The guy who'd been shot three times was the younger of the two. His name was Reggie, and according to the police, he'd been dancing with a girl who may or may not have been romantically involved with the shooter. When the shooter asked the younger brother to step aside, words were exchanged, the older brother, Greg, jumped in, and a fight broke out. Then the shooter disappeared, only to return just before the club closed. Reggie was still dancing with the shooter's girl-friend—or the woman he *wanted* to be his girlfriend—and the shooter approached them, got in Reggie's face, pulled out a gun, and fired. Greg had evidently seen the situation unfolding and jumped in front of the gun. He caught the first bullet in his abdomen, and the shooter kept firing, striking Reggie three times. Everyone in the club ran for cover, and the shooter fled. He was still on the run, but the police seemed confident they would find him, the chief resident said.

The details of the story jolted my memory. I suddenly recalled what the young woman had said as she helped Greg into the hospital: "He tried to save his life." Her words, lost in the pandemonium, now made sense. I imagined the chaos in the club: patrons screaming, ducking under tables, trampling one another in their scramble to get away.

I was reminded of a night during medical school when I got jumped by a group of New Brunswick dudes at a popular off-campus club, the Down Under.

"Where you been?" someone had shouted as I arrived, late, with three of my college friends. "This party is blazing!"

I started dancing without a partner, then spotted one of my homegirls dancing with a guy I didn't know. For some reason (probably the beer), I moved onto the dance floor with her. Mistake number one. That's a huge no-no in club etiquette, a show of disrespect to her partner. The dude glared at me, letting me know this wasn't over. I ignored him as he walked off the dance floor and disappeared. I was still dancing with her when I saw him return with a few guys and point in my direction. I played it cool, finished the song, gave my friend a hug, and moved around the club, letting my boys know something was about to go down.

How ridiculous it all seems to me now.

Sure enough, when the party ended and I stepped out of the club, eight or nine dudes swooped in, punching and kicking me. The New Brunswick locals didn't care too much for Rutgers college boys invading their space. Somehow I was able to look up, and there was Rameck rushing into the fray, throwing punches, pulling guys off me. Then came our friend Sean, wielding a huge board that he'd picked up somewhere, charging into the ruckus, plucking off the locals. I was in an armlock, tussling with another guy when we spun into a huge storefront window, which shattered. The two of us fell through it and landed, still throwing punches, on the bed of broken glass. Seconds later, the New Brunswick police were on the scene, and the crowd scattered. The local boys got away. I was thrown against the police car and frisked, while trying to explain that I'd been jumped. Fortunately, a few people from the crowd corroborated my story, and the officers let Rameck and me go. They handcuffed Sean and arrested him for using the board as a weapon. We were able to scrape together enough money to bail him out. Many years later, a routine dental exam revealed that Rameck had suffered a fractured jaw, which he presumed had happened during the brawl and which somehow managed to heal on its own without displacement.

All three of us were fortunate to walk away that night with just one cracked jaw and a few cuts and bruises among us. I couldn't imagine the guilt I would have carried if one of my boys had lost his life over something so trivial. Yet this scenario plays out far too often in nightclubs throughout the country. Tempers, fueled by alcohol, explode over the smallest perceived insult—a wrong look, a stepped-on shoe, rejection from a beautiful woman—suddenly throwing everything into chaos. Add guns to the mix, and many times someone winds up dead. This kind of incident actually appears to be growing more common, particularly in urban centers, according to some experts who have studied the issue.

"The violence in nightclubs and bars across the country has increased dramatically," Robert Smith, a San Diego consultant who specializes in nightclub crime, told the *Sun-Sentinel* in Florida in a story published in February 2012. "It's not just in your town, it's nationwide."

Instead of solving problems with their fists, people are carrying guns, Smith said.

In the same article, Tammy Anderson, a sociology professor at the University of Delaware, told the newspaper that after studying nightclub violence, she had concluded that one of the common elements of the brawls was "macho posturing." Men try to show off their toughness and physical prowess to attract women, which can escalate their response to the most innocent bump or minor exchange of words. "Those personal affronts become catalysts for violent offending and victimization," she said.

Several cities have passed laws trying to crack down on such violence. In 2007, for example, the New York City Council passed measures requiring security cameras at the entrances and exits of dozens of bars and clubs. It gave the city the power to shut down businesses selling fake identification cards, as well as those that hire unlicensed bouncers. Such measures can be helpful, but nothing is a replacement for personal vigilance and responsibility.

I knew from the moment I stepped onto the dance floor with my homegirl at the nightclub that my actions would piss off her dance partner. I just didn't care. But if I'd taken a few extra seconds to consider the consequences, I might have made a different choice.

After the morning report, my team, Trauma A, checked in on all the patients remaining from our previous shift. When we got to the Surgical Intensive Care Unit and made it to Greg's room, I saw a familiar face. It was the girl who'd helped him into the emergency department. I introduced myself, and she remembered me. She was Tara, his girlfriend. I told her I was sorry to hear what had happened. I was sure she had been in touch with the police officers investigating the incident, but she was eager to know if I'd heard anything more.

"Did they catch him yet?" Tara asked, referring to the shooter. "They have his girlfriend. I can't understand what's taking so long."

I told her that I hadn't heard anything new.

"Dr. Davis, Greg always looked after Reggie," she continued. "Their mother made sure they always took care of each other. She would tell them both, 'All you have is each other.'"

That bond had held tight. I had to finish my rounds with the rest of the team, and so I assured Tara that I would return later. But I hadn't had a chance to make it back when I heard a Code Blue call from the Surgical Intensive Care Unit—a cardiac arrest. I dropped the note I was writing about another patient, grabbed my stethoscope, and sprinted over. I reached in my back pocket for gloves. I always kept a spare pair or two on me since they sometimes weren't readily available when I needed them.

As I barged through the door, my gut told me it would be Greg. The unit had a dozen beds, all critical patients, but he was by far the most critical that day. And, in fact, the junior resident was standing over Greg, supervising his care. One of the nurses was performing chest compressions. I stepped in quickly to take over. This was my expertise. I knew the medical side of a cardiac arrest. Epinephrine was pushed, followed by atropine. After administering several rounds, we eyed the monitor and felt for a pulse in his leg. The femoral artery didn't give way to any thumping. I felt no rhythm under my finger. There was no heartbeat coming through the stethoscope, and the monitor showed a flat line. At just twenty-three years old, Greg was dead.

Tara, who'd been so tough until now, broke down, screaming and crying. For the rest of the day, Greg's grieving family came and went. I was called to the room several times to talk to new family members. His death was still so shocking that each one wanted details. They'd thought he'd survived the worst of it. How had this happened? I didn't mind spending as much time as I could with them. It was the least I could do. Before the family left the hospital, the brothers' mother led us all in a prayer. She prayed for her sons and for the protection of her family. She asked the Lord to forgive her boys for whatever role they may have played in the brawl and to protect and guide Greg's soul.

"Amen," we said in unison.

Long after they'd all gone home, Greg was still on my mind. His life had been snuffed out for what? Because some dude felt disrespected that his girl was dancing with someone else? Pride could be deadly.

A few days after Greg's death, I was walking past Reggie's room and decided to check on him. I knocked softly, simultaneously pushed the door open, and stuck my head in. He was sitting up, staring into space. He appeared to be deep in thought and never even seemed to notice that I was there, and so I left him alone. A couple of days later, I tried again. He was sitting up and watching television while eating lunch. The breathing tube in his throat was gone, and he was recovering well from the gunshot wounds. I remembered those larger-than-life bullet holes he and Greg had had. A high-caliber gun must have been used at close range. Reggie's lungs were showing promising signs of recovery, which meant his chest tube would soon be pulled. And there was no paralysis. "Good morning," I said, making my way over to him. "I'm Dr. Davis. How's your breathing?"

Without looking my way, he murmured, "It's okay. I feel better today than yesterday."

"That's what we were hoping for," I responded. "You'll have an X-ray later to check on your lungs. If all is well, then I'll pull that tube out of your chest."

Reggie nodded, still focused on the television. Highlights from the Lakers game were on. The team was on the road to the playoffs and had taken a beating the night before. Also a basketball fan, I saw an instant opportunity to connect and commented on the loss. Reggie dropped his head, as if he was still in disbelief over his team's performance. His icy demeanor began to thaw.

"Man, if Kobe and Shaq could only have gotten along, the Lakers would have won ten championships," he said.

My eyes turned to the TV. "How can you like the Lakers? We're here in New Jersey," I teased.

Reggie smiled for the first time since I'd entered the room. "Doc, the Nets make it hard to like them."

I couldn't argue with that. I had been a Lakers fan in the eighties when Magic and Kareem were playing. Together, Shaq and Kobe seemed to bring back some of that eighties magic to the Lakers, but egos were starting to get in the way. After the Lakers won the 2000 championship, the two stars engaged in a nasty public feud, each trying to one-up the other. They would still lead their team to two more back-to-back championships—the famous "three-peat"—but fans of the game suspected that a breakup was inevitable long before it actually happened. That would come to pass three years later with Shaq's trade to the Miami Heat.

"I'm telling you, the Lakers would have won as many rings as Bill Russell," Reggie said, referring to the former Boston Celtics star who led his team to an astonishing eleven championships. "I'm telling you, Doc, it would have happened."

I gave him a skeptical look. "Man, today's players don't stick it out with one another that long. After a championship or two, the stars are off to the next team or holding out for the salary demands."

Reggie paused and then added: "That wouldn't be me and Greg. If we were on that team, we would show those guys how it's done. We checked our egos at the door. We would have won eleven rings. We always took care of each other."

I smiled. "Now, that's what's up. If we had more guys with that attitude, we would be better off."

I sensed that Reggie was beginning to drop his defenses a bit, maybe realizing that the hospital was neutral ground. It was nice to see him in good spirits. But what came next surprised me.

"Doc, I miss my brother," he said. "We would always watch the games together. He was shot the same night I was."

"I remember your brother," I said. "I took care of both of you the night of the shooting."

This was the first time that Reggie had opened up to anyone about his brother or the shooting. When a social worker had visited previously, Reggie wouldn't say a word.

"This experience has changed my life," he whispered. "Things will never be the same. Doc, I still can't believe that he jumped in front of the bullet. I can't believe that he would risk his life that way. If he'd stayed in the background, he would be here talking to me. Yeah, I still would have been shot, but I wouldn't have to live with his death on my conscience. He's—" Reggie broke off, and paused for a painful second and corrected himself. "He *was* my best friend."

The pain and guilt were palpable.

"Don't be hard on yourself, man," I said. "It wasn't your fault." I reminded him that he wasn't the one who'd pulled the trigger, and that his older brother felt a sense of responsibility for him and wouldn't want him moping around feeling depressed.

I felt I was connecting with him, so I kept pushing. "You know, there is something to be learned here."

He stared at me. "Yeah, I know." He was wearing outdated, brown plastic-rimmed glasses, which made him look more mature than his years. "All I was doing was dancing with some girl, and her dude got all beside himself," Reggie began. "As soon as I saw him come back into the bar, I should have known that it was going to go down. That's my fault. I slipped."

He seemed to need to talk, so I just kept quiet and listened.

"All I remember is my brother pushing me out of the way, and then there were flashes of light. I heard people screaming and at the same time I felt a burning sensation in my chest. That was it. I passed out. I would give anything just to have my brother here."

I placed my hand on his shoulder. "I know, Reggie. I know," I told him. "Take it one day at a time and keep moving forward, with the thought of Greg watching over you." Then I wished him well and left the room.

Sometime later the shooter surrendered and was eventually sentenced to life in prison. I was glad that Greg's family got the justice they sought, yet I couldn't forget that from one frivolous encounter on a nightclub dance floor, two young men's lives had been lost— one to death and the other to jail. And still another one would be haunted forever.

8

THE FEAR FACTOR

My landlady, Mrs. Jackson, had become my second mother. She ran a small home-based daycare center and had touched so many lives with her warmth and nurturing manner that her former preschool children returned to visit long after they had left her home. She had what I joked was her own tribe of men and women, all ages, who were always stopping by to check on her. I'd already become one of them. My plan had been to live in her house for three months while I got on my feet financially, but my time there kept expanding. Little did I know then that I would stay on Hazelwood Avenue for six years.

The Christmas holidays were approaching in 2001 when I noticed Mrs. Jackson hobbling around the house on a bad knee. She hadn't fallen and couldn't remember bumping into anything—she just woke up one morning, and it was swollen and sore.

"Must be my arthritis," she said, leaning on the big black umbrella she was using as a cane. I suspected that was the case, too, but I suggested she come to the hospital so I could get a specialist to check it out, just to be sure. But she refused. Like most busy moms, Mrs. Jackson put everyone else first. She rarely took time away from the kids, even to go to the doctor for a routine checkup. "I have to be here for my babies and their moms," she insisted. "What would they do if the daycare was closed?"

For two weeks after the pain started, she simply "rubbed the knee down," with this potion or that one, limping, hurting, hoping it would get better. Even with a doctor living in her house, she preferred diagnosing herself, treating practically every ailment with one of her home remedies—specially brewed teas for coughs and sore throats, strong-smelling ointments to break up chest congestion or soothe aching joints. I even offered to make an appointment for her, but she kept putting me off.

"Don't worry, it will get better," she said.

"It might be arthritis, but it might not be," I warned.

Finally, Mrs. Jackson agreed to come to Beth Israel for tests. It was Christmas Eve day, so her "babies" were home with their families, and she assumed the emergency room wouldn't be as crowded as usual.

As soon as I reported to work that morning, I phoned the rheumatologist on duty and asked if she could take a look at my "other mother" in the emergency department. As a favor to me, my colleague agreed, and I called Mrs. Jackson to let her know that she needed to get to the hospital right away. Within a half hour, she was being examined. The diagnosis: She had excessive fluid in her joints. The doctor then performed an arthrocentesis, a joint aspiration using a needle to drain the fluid from the knee. After removing about fifty milliliters of yellowish liquid, the doctor injected the knee with steroids and an anesthetic, which would help relieve the pain. Afterward, I sent Mrs. Jackson for an X-ray to confirm that there were no fractures or other bone damage, and she rewarded me with a huge smile. She said she felt better than she had in weeks. I finished the paperwork for her release, handed her a prescription for pain, and told her I'd get her an appointment with the joint specialist to figure out what had caused the fluid buildup. Now she beamed like a proud parent.

"Sam, I'm glad you made me come," she said, as I walked her

toward the hospital exit, where her daughter was waiting for her. "I never would have done this on my own. Don't get stuck here for Christmas, now. You know I'll have dinner at home."

For me, Christmas had come a day early. Mrs. Jackson had allowed me to take care of her, and that was a wonderful, unexpected gift.

Unfortunately, Mrs. Jackson's reluctance to see a doctor isn't unusual. I treat many patients whose busy lives or fear of doctors prevent them from seeking much-needed medical care right away. In 2003, I witnessed one of the worst examples of what can happen when a man I'll call Mr. Tate showed up during my shift at Irvington General, another big-city medical center that is part of Beth Israel's training network. As I passed through the emergency department on my way to the doctor's call room one day, I noticed him sitting in one of the examining rooms, head down, hands folded in his lap, waiting patiently to see a doctor. Next to him stood a much younger woman—his daughter, I presumed—with an agitated look on her face. I made it to the call room, set my bag on the old metal desk, and pulled out my stethoscope, rubber hammer, pen light, and lunch. I found a spot in the refrigerator for my chicken salad sandwich and hoped it wouldn't suddenly grow legs and walk away. On more than one occasion my lunch had mysteriously disappeared from the community fridge. That accomplished, I headed back to the emergency department, where I picked up some charts and began forming a mental game plan: How many patients were waiting? Who would I see next? Who was the most critical? I was counting patients in my head when an irritated voice interrupted my thoughts.

"Can you *puh-leeze* hurry up and see my father?"

I looked up to see the young woman who had been standing next to the elderly man in room 5. I'm certain my face told her I didn't appreciate the ambush, but I knew I'd get an earful from the hospital administration if I voiced the words that came to mind. I held my tongue, placed my blue stethoscope—the same one I'd had since medical school—around my neck, pulled the patient's chart, and followed her. On the way, I scanned the man's information. The first thing that jumped out at me was his age. When I'd walked by earlier, he'd seemed to be a frail, elderly man of at least seventy, but now I saw I was off—way off. The age printed on the chart was fifty-five. He was complaining of throat pain, a sore tongue, and swelling on the left side of his neck. The nurse triage sheet noted that he had been seen a week earlier at another hospital. It appeared he had been diagnosed with a throat infection, given a prescription for antibiotics, and sent home.

"Hi," I said, extending my hand. "I'm Dr. Davis. How are you doing today?"

"I'm doing great," he said, introducing himself. He had a smoker's voice, raspy and dry.

He'd been suffering with the same symptoms for a year, he told me, and the medicines he'd been given at the other hospital a week ago hadn't worked a bit. His daughter, Michelle, handed me a worn brown paper bag with two empty pill bottles, one for penicillin, the other for ibuprofen.

These were the right medications for a throat infection, I thought to myself. Before I could even note the medications on my chart, Michelle was on the attack: "Look, you *better* do something!" she snapped. "He's sick, and these so-called medicines ain't working! The other doctor said these would make him better, and they clearly haven't."

Her voice was raised, her eyebrows were wrinkled, her nostrils flared, and her right index finger waved in the air for added effect. Michelle was only a few inches shorter than me and built like a high school football player, with a certain swagger. But it was important for me to stay calm. A nurse, apparently hearing Michelle's raised voice, peeked into the room to make sure everything was okay. I signaled to her that I had it under control.

"Why is it so slow here?" Michelle continued. "We've been here for hours and nothing's been done to help us."

"I understand your frustration," I said calmly, then turned to her father and asked about his medical history. He told me that although his throat had been bothering him for around a year, the symptoms had worsened in the week since his previous hospital visit. He had no medical insurance, but his daughter had insisted he go to another hospital, this time Irvington General.

"You say you've had throat pain for about a year?" I asked, trying to make sure I'd understood correctly.

"That's right. It comes and goes, but lately it's been here all the time."

"Do you smoke?"

Mr. Tate nodded yes.

"Do you drink?"

"Well, Doc, I used to drink in my twenties and thirties, but not anymore, especially since my throat has been bothering me. I'm trying to quit smoking, too."

"How many cigarettes would you say you smoke a day now?"

"About three, but I used to smoke maybe a pack, a pack and a half."

Michelle interrupted: "Stop lying, Daddy. You still smoke a whole pack."

I continued my line of questioning: "Have you experienced any weight loss?"

"Yes," he said reticently. "I have."

Throat pain off and on for a year. Weight loss. Swelling on the side of his neck. My concern was growing.

"Dr. Davis, I think I'm losing weight because I can't eat. It's the pain in my throat that's causing all of this. It hurts a lot. Believe me, if it wasn't for the pain, I wouldn't be here. I hate coming to these hospitals. You doctors always want to cut somebody, and you always talk over patients' heads, like we understand all that fancy medical talk."

I promised him I would do my best to be clear and make sure he understood everything that was going on. "If you have any questions at all, don't hesitate to ask," I said.

"I'm just afraid you're gonna tell me something I don't want to hear . . . And whatever it is, there is no way in the world I'm going to allow you to cut me," he added. "See, I'm okay with whatever happens. I've lived my life. I take my herbal medicines and pray. That's what I believe in, and that's all I need."

It saddened me that at age fifty-five, Mr. Tate thought he'd lived a full life and was ready to give up. How had any doctor diagnosed him with just a throat infection without doing further tests? Either the doctor hadn't bothered to look at him closely or had simply instructed him to follow up with his primary physician. I hoped Mr. Tate's lack of medical insurance, his distrust of the system, or his lack of understanding hadn't caused the other doctor to just dismiss him without the same care that may have been provided to a better educated, better insured customer. I had my suspicions, though.

"Don't worry," I said. "I have no plans to cut anyone who doesn't need surgery, and I'm not here to try to alter your beliefs."

He eyed me suspiciously. "They sure are making you doctors younger and younger," he said. "I hope you don't think that I'm a guinea pig or something."

Guinea pig—I'd heard that term many times from black men and women of Mr. Tate's generation, and they were only half kidding. Many of them were old enough to remember hearing in 1972 about the infamous government-sanctioned syphilis experiment at the Tuskegee Institute, a historically black college. The U.S. Public Health Service was rocked by scandal when it came to light that its doctors, working with Tuskegee, had in the 1930s recruited 600 sharecroppers from Macon County, Alabama—399 who were already infected with syphilis and 201 who were not—for a study of the progression of the disease in black men. To the participants, who were poor and mostly illiterate, the offer to receive free medical treatment for "bad blood"—a term that the local black residents often used to refer to a variety of illnesses from anemia to venereal diseases—must have seemed like a stroke of good fortune. After all, they were also promised a hot meal on their days at the clinic, free medical exams, free treatment for minor ailments, free transportation to the clinic, and free burial benefits. But the participants were never told that they had syphilis. Even worse, they were denied treatment when penicillin became widely available in 1947 as a safe and effective cure. The study was finally forced to shut down in 1972 when newspapers broke the news. By then, just 74 of the original 399 men were still alive, and massive damage had been done. Twenty-eight of the men had died of syphilis, another hundred had died from related complications, forty of their wives had been infected, and nineteen of their children had been born with congenital syphilis. The fear that resulted from this abuse by the medical establishment has reverberated among African Americans ever since.

A similar but lesser-known controversy erupted in more recent years when syphilis experiments by U.S. doctors in Guatemala between 1946 and 1948 were exposed. As part of that study, doctors deliberately infected nearly 700 prisoners, soldiers, and mental patients with syphilis (and in some instances gonorrhea). Some Guatemalan health officials approved the study, but none of the patients gave their consent. The Guatemalan study was supervised by Dr. John Charles Cutler, a Public Health Service researcher and former assistant surgeon general who was also involved with the Tuskegee experiment in the 1960s. In October 2010, the U.S. government officially apologized to Guatemala for the controversial study.

The more well-known Tuskegee experiment is often cited by medical professionals as the primary reason that minorities still fear the medical establishment and are underrepresented in clinical trials for new medications and treatments, as well as in bone marrow, organ, and blood donations. Some minorities even believe that HIV is disproportionately high in African American communities because it is actually man-made and was part of some kind of deliberate extermination plot.

Though the fear and conspiracy theories still linger, there are hopeful signs that the passage of time has begun to change things for the better. In November 2006, the *Journal of Health Care for the Poor and Underserved* published the results of a survey entitled "The Tuskegee Legacy Project: Willingness of Minorities to Participate in Biomedical Research," which questioned 1,133 black, white, and Hispanic adults about their possible participation in medical research and their associated fears. The survey showed no measurable difference by race in participants' willingness to participate in medical research. However, black men and women were nearly twice as likely to report the fear of being used as a "guinea pig."

I had no idea whether Mr. Tate knew anything about the Tuskegee experiment, but his fear was real. It had kept him from seeking help when his symptoms first appeared, and now I dreaded what the result of that might be. I did my best to reassure him that my only intention was to discover the source of his pain and help him feel better.

"Mr. Tate, I'm here to help," I said. "You remind me of my father, and I'll give you the same care that I'd give him."

With a tongue blade in my hand, I asked him to open his mouth. I took a look at his teeth, gums, and the back of his throat. As soon as he said "Ahh," I could see that the entire left border of his tongue was eroded. It appeared as if small bites had been nibbled out, and the color had changed from pink to dark brownish red. Next, I examined his neck. There, I felt a hard, golf ball–sized lump to the left of his Adam's apple.

"Okay, we need to order some tests," I said. I spoke slowly and clearly. It was important to me that he fully understood the steps we were about to take.

"What do you think is going on?" he asked, his eyes probing mine for answers.

"I'm not totally sure," I responded. "That's why we need to order the tests."

Mr. Tate sighed; it sounded as if air was being let out of a balloon. "There you go. You doctors always want to find a way to drive up the bill. I don't want any tests."

Michelle, who to my amazement had been entirely quiet for the last several minutes, chimed in: "Can't you just give him some medicine that works, so we can get out of here?"

"I assure you the tests are necessary," I said, writing on his chart my orders for blood work and a radiology study. "It's the only way to find out exactly what's going on. I understand your situation and I certainly don't want to waste your time."

Mr. Tate nodded reluctantly.

I left the room and asked the clerk to put in an order for a CAT scan of Mr. Tate's neck. (Most people are more familiar with X-rays. By comparison, if an X-ray is like regular TV, a CAT scan is high-definition TV. It allows doctors to visualize the bones, muscles, blood vessels, and any abnormalities of a body part. In Mr. Tate's case, I was hoping the CAT scan would reveal the source of the lump.) When I returned to the room, Mr. Tate was sitting on the stretcher, and Michelle was pacing. Both looked intense and worried.

"You'll be going over to radiology very shortly," I said, trying my best to explain things simply and keep him informed at every step.

It wasn't long before an orderly arrived with a wheelchair to take Mr. Tate for the scan. The study was completed in about twenty minutes, and I noticed him in the hallway as he was being wheeled back to the department.

"Hey, you're back," I said. "How did it go?"

"Not bad," he responded. "It was quicker than I thought. How long before you have my results?"

"Not long. I have to wait for the radiologist, the doctor who reads the films, to take a look. But I'll let you know as soon as I hear."

"Okay, then."

Half an hour later, the results began coming through the fax machine. I'd prayed my suspicion was wrong. Unfortunately, it wasn't.

The paper read: "Cancerous necrotic lymph nodes."

The cancer had probably spread from the vocal cord area of his throat and now involved the mouth and lymph nodes, too, which explained the raspy voice. The poor guy most likely had been living with it for a while. In a way, my job was done. I had discovered what was wrong. But for him, the ordeal was just beginning. I dreaded breaking the news to them. Moving slowly to room 5, I thought to myself, *This isn't what I signed up for when I decided to go to medical school.*

Once inside the room, I moved toward the familiar worn green chair in the corner, deliberately avoiding eye contact with both Mr. Tate and Michelle. I had to take a seat for this one.

"Okay, I have your results," I said.

Mr. Tate looked up, and I stared directly into his sunken eyes. At this stage it's always better to come right out and say it, instead of prolonging the agony. "I'm sorry, Mr. Tate, but the CAT scan shows a very progressive form of throat cancer."

There. I'd said it. Now I steeled myself for one of the most difficult parts of delivering this kind of news: the patient's reaction.

Silence followed. The news had knocked the wind out of Michelle for a second. She screamed and then looked at me with a mix of fear and anger. She seemed to be trying to process the diagnosis: "What does that mean?"

Mr. Tate immediately diverted his attention to her. "Sweetie, don't worry. I'm going to be all right."

"No, Daddy, I want to know!"

I was amazed. The man had been hit with the worst news of his life, and his first reaction was to comfort his daughter. Michelle took a deep breath and asked again, more calmly: "What does all of this mean?"

I began to explain, "The treatment—"

She cut me off: "Is my daddy gonna die?"

The question stunned me, but I should have guessed she would be direct.

"Well, as I was about to say, the treatment for this kind of cancer is a tracheotomy and an artificial voice box, along with both radiation and chemotherapy to manage the tumor. It is somewhat difficult to estimate how long your father has to live. Depending on the stage of the tumor, it can range from months to years. I have to be candid with you. I believe that due to the mouth and lymph node involvement, the cancer has already spread, which isn't a promising sign. At this stage, his life expectancy depends on how well he responds to treatment."

"You still haven't answered my question," Michelle persisted. "What I'm asking is, is my father going to die?"

I never like playing God, telling a terminally ill patient or that patient's loved ones how much time is left. I've seen patients live far beyond any of the experts' time estimates, and I've seen others die when I thought they would live. But I also believe that my patients deserve to know as much as I can tell them about what they are facing.

"Not immediately," I responded. "My best guess is that he has a year or two, maybe three. But no one can say for sure."

Michelle wiped her tears. "My God, Daddy, why didn't I bring you sooner?"

"Baby, you know how I feel about hospitals and doctors," he answered. "Plus, I don't have insurance, and I already depend on you too much. It isn't your fault."

Something exploded in my mind. I was suddenly furious. America, a nation with incomprehensible wealth, did not provide affordable healthcare for everyone—an issue that the administration of President Barack Obama has fought hard to address. While there are free community-based clinics, the demand so exceeds the need that patients sometimes have to wait upward of six months for an appointment. Mr. Tate was dying for many reasons; his lack of medical insurance shouldn't have been one of them. The man hadn't been to a doctor in years. His cancer most likely would have been detected earlier if he had been under the care of a primary doctor. But his fear of doctors, coupled with his lack of insurance, had stood in the way of him getting the help he needed. Of course, his smoking habit didn't help either. But my guess is that there weren't too many people around him who enforced the need for him to stop. That's a doctor's job; that's my job. At this stage, though, the damage had been done, and it was irreversible.

I rose from my chair. It was time for me to move on and hand Mr. Tate's care over to others: surgeons, oncologists, counselors. "Is there anything I can do for you, Mr. Tate?"

"No," he replied.

"Okay, you'll need to stay in the hospital." I wanted him to be seen as soon as possible by cancer specialists so that he could begin receiving the appropriate treatment.

"I'll put your chart in for admission," I added. "I hope we can get you a room tonight."

Overcrowding is always an issue, so a room was not guaranteed that night. I've admitted patients who ended up spending several nights in the emergency department waiting for a room assignment. Some were even treated for their medical problems and discharged without ever making it to a hospital room. Back at the desk, I asked the clerk to begin arranging for Mr. Tate's admission. If no bed was available, I was sure he would sign out, and there was a good chance we would never see him again. I stuck around to make sure he was assigned a room. As simple as it seemed, getting that room meant everything to me in that moment.

Once I was sure about the room, I returned to share the news with Mr. Tate. But just as I was about to step into the room where they were waiting, I saw the formerly tough, hurried Michelle curled up on the narrow stretcher beside her father. Her head rested on his shoulder, and she lay silently in his arms. I couldn't interrupt the tender moment, and so I backed out of the room. A picture of my own father flashed through my mind.

Pop was being treated for prostate cancer. He had remarried in 1987 and retired four years later, after thirty-five years of fueling planes at Butler Aviation. In the late 1990s, he and his wife, Thelma, moved to Raleigh, North Carolina, after she retired. Pop and I had stayed in touch through telephone calls and periodic visits, and I usually remembered to send birthday and Father's Day cards. But I had trouble making an emotional connection with him. He was from that stoic, ironclad generation of men who possessed an external toughness that blocked access to any soft spots or tender feelings on the inside. He had continued to provide the basics, food and shelter, paying off the mortgage on our Ludlow Street house a month at a time, long after he left. But I'd felt abandoned. I was twelve when he and my mother divorced, leaving me to fend for myself through the turbulent teen years and into manhood in a decaying neighborhood overtaken by the 1980s crack epidemic.

Pop did show up for the big moments, though. He was there for practically every visitation opportunity during the four weeks I spent in juvenile detention—but by then I'd developed the hardened exterior of the guys on the streets and could only sit with him in awkward silence. He was there, too, beaming, at the graduations and award ceremonies. But our interactions always seemed distant, more businesslike than personal, even in my teenage years when he scooped me up for an occasional night out at McDonald's or the time in college when he forked over $2,000 to help me buy my used Honda Accord. Showing up and helping out financially were the only ways he knew to express his pride and love. I appreciated it and at times even sent him greeting cards that told him he was the most wonderful father in the world. But that sentiment always seemed to compete with the anger and resentment I felt inside. Like any kid, I longed to hear the words that he could never bring himself to say: "I love you," "I'm proud of you."

After his cancer diagnosis in 2003, Thelma called to break the news, and the three of us discussed his treatment options. He decided to pursue radiation therapy, and Thelma was diligent in informing me about his health. She kept meticulous records of his doctor visits and made sure he got to all of his appointments on time. I can say with certainty that my father followed his treatment regimen faithfully because of her . . . and that he trusted medicine because of me. Whenever his doctors introduced a new medicine or therapy or tried to explain something he didn't understand, he told them, "Make sure you give my son a call. You know he's a doctor, too." I felt his confidence and pride in me every time he asked for my advice and surrendered: "Whatever you say, I'll do."

Years after his diagnosis, I would learn about my father's childhood for the first time. I don't know why it had never come up before then; we just didn't have that kind of sharing relationship. I would learn that he was just a boy—not quite ten years old—when his own father died, leaving him, too, to navigate manhood alone. That bit of knowledge would go a long way toward helping me begin to understand and forgive my pop. But in the meantime, I just knew that I loved him. And there were moments when, even as a grown man with a slew of degrees and honors, I still yearned for a close bond with him.

As I backed out of Mr. Tate's room that day, I made a mental note to call my pop, just because.

Prostate Cancer

Prostate cancer is the most common cancer among men, regardless of race or ethnicity. It is more common among African American men than men of other races, and black men are more likely to die from it than other men. Some men have no symptoms, which is why it is important to have a yearly checkup. The symptoms include:

- Difficulty starting urination
- Weak or interrupted flow of urine
- Frequent urination, especially at night
- Difficulty emptying the bladder completely
- Pain or burning during urination
- Blood in the urine or semen
- Pain in the back, hips, or pelvis that doesn't go away
- Painful ejaculation

*The above symptoms may be caused by conditions other than prostate cancer; if you have symptoms that concern you, see your doctor.

Smoking and Death

- The adverse health effects of smoking account for nearly one of every five deaths each year in the United States.
- More deaths are caused each year by tobacco use than by human immunodeficiency virus (HIV), illegal drug use, alcohol use, motor vehicle injuries, suicides, and murders combined.
- Smoking causes an estimated 90 percent of all lung cancer deaths in men and 80 percent of all lung cancer deaths in women.
- An estimated 90 percent of all deaths from chronic obstructive lung disease are caused by smoking.
- Smoking causes the following cancers:
  - Acute myeloid leukemia
  - Bladder cancer

- Cancer of the cervix
- Cancer of the esophagus
- Kidney cancer
- Cancer of the larynx (voice box)
- Lung cancer
- Cancer of the oral cavity (mouth)
- Pancreatic cancer
- Cancer of the pharynx (throat)
- Stomach cancer

For help with quitting smoking: 1-800-Quit-Now (1-800-784-8669); TTY 1-800-332-8615

Source: The Centers for Disease Control and Prevention

9

THE FISH BOWL

The closest thing to an office I had at the hospital was a tiny shared space we staffers called the "Fish Bowl." It wasn't exactly what I had in mind when I finished medical school. Instead of a nice place where I could hang my hard-earned diplomas, certificates, awards, and family photos, my workspace was an overcrowded room I shared with other staff, located in the center of the emergency department. The largest wall was a window that offered a panoramic view of the jam-packed waiting area, examining rooms, and hallway. The patients could look in at us, and we could look out at them—thus, its name, the Fish Bowl.

The Fish Bowl was the E.R.'s nerve center. Three or four staffers could fit comfortably in the room under normal circumstances, but two or three times as many doctors, nurses, technicians, and aides were regularly squeezed in there most days, consulting about a patient, talking on the phone, printing a chart, writing a prescription, or waiting for one of the room's four computers. (There was always a waiting line at the door for the computers.)

In an effort to deal with the crowding, the department was always undergoing renovation. As soon as one project was completed, the architect was called back to plan the next expansion. Still, our department couldn't keep up with the demand for more space. Hospitals throughout the country faced the same challenge. Population growth and increasing numbers of seniors (the group most likely to seek ambulatory care) have caused a surge in emergency room visits nationwide since the mid-1990s. From 1997 to 2007, trips to the E.R. jumped from 95 million to 117 million, an increase of about 23 percent, according to federal records. At the same time, hospitals and emergency departments have been closing in dramatic numbers, particularly in urban areas and suburbs with largely low-income, non-white populations. And the situation threatens to grow even more critical as the Baby Boomers continue to age.

For doctors and nurses, the overcrowded conditions have meant greatly increased nightly caseloads and little time to spend with patients. I often saw Linda, one of my favorite nurses, distributing medications, changing urine Foleys, placing a patient on a monitor, drawing blood, running among as many as ten patients, rarely stopping for even a bathroom break or meal during her entire twelve-hour shift. This behind-the-scenes stress is, of course, mostly invisible to patients, who are often cranky by the time I meet them—and understandably so. It's bad enough that they have to experience the emergency that landed them in the E.R. in the first place, but then they have to wait an hour or two to see a doctor; and if they happen to arrive when crowding is at its peak, they may end up being treated in a converted hallway with merely a thin curtain separating them and their private business from fellow patients.

At times, when the emergency department and hospital are filled to capacity, we are placed on "divert status," which means hospitals are not allowed to accept another patient brought in by ambulance, except in life-threatening cases. The rule doesn't matter, though, because the emergency medical technicians still drive right up to our doors with familiar excuses: "The patient demanded to come here," or "Every other hospital is on divert as well."

There we were one day, crowded in the Fish Bowl on divert status. Operations in the emergency department had come almost to a standstill as we waited for the traffic jam to clear, so my colleagues and I sat around and talked. One of them was planning her wedding and couldn't decide whether to have the ceremony in Hawaii, Jamaica, Fiji, or New York. A resident sitting at one of the computers chimed in, offering another suggestion: "Turks and Caicos." He brought up dozens of photos on the computer of him, his new wife, and the wedding they'd had there to show us. The conversation piqued my interest. I'd begun to travel a bit in my free time since med school; whenever I saved up enough money for a vacation, I tried to land on a beach somewhere—in California, Cancún, Jamaica, Saint Martin, Puerto Rico, Belize. I couldn't take my eyes off the beautiful scenery of the Turks and Caicos Islands in one photo after another. I could hardly believe that this paradise existed just two-and-a-half hours from New York by plane.

From the corner of my eye, I noticed Nurse Linda rush past, leading four patients from the waiting room to the examining rooms. That meant others must have been discharged and the pace was about to pick up again. I moved to the doorway and took one last peek at my colleague's wedding photos. Just then, I felt a light tap on my shoulder from outside the door. I turned and saw a familiar face.

"Rick?" I said, extending my hand to a friend from my old neighborhood. "What's up, man? I haven't seen you in years. How's everything?"

His appearance told me that the years had not been kind. He responded with a half-crooked smile, revealing more missing teeth than good ones.

"I'm good," he said.

"What brings you here? Everything all right?"

He pointed to the waiting room. I looked out through the Fish Bowl window and saw a vaguely familiar face. For a moment I tried to remember where I'd met the haggard old guy sitting out there. "Yeah, that's Tony," Rick answered, noticing my bewilderment.

I was too stunned even to speak.

"I saw him walking the street," Rick continued. "I couldn't believe it myself. He's homeless. I think he's using drugs, too. At least that's what they're saying in the streets. You know I had to help. I couldn't leave him out there. Marshall, you know Tony. He was never this way. Ever since we were kids he always had it together."

"Yeah, I know," I responded.

Tony and I had grown up on the same block, and our mothers were friends. The two of them often went shopping together or worked outside at the same time, shoveling snow or raking leaves, while Tony and I played in one of our backyards. We were in the same grade, had the same teachers, and spent countless hours playing together after school. We borrowed each other's video games and played basketball in his backyard until it was so dark we could barely see the ball. It was Tony, not my father, who taught me to ride a bike. I was ten years old, well past the age when most kids learned, and I was embarrassed. I'd even lied about it, telling friends I knew how to ride. It was easy enough to get away with the lie since I didn't have a bicycle. But the excuses kept getting tougher every time one of the kids in the neighborhood offered to let me borrow his bike to prove my skills.

One July night, Tony handed me his bike, and I just stood there, staring at it. He recognized my shame and said simply, "I'll show you." He held the back of the bike and ran alongside as I pedaled. Because it was so hot inside the house during summer, Moms allowed me to stay outside later than usual, as long as I didn't stray too far. All night long, I pedaled up and down the block with Tony in tow, at first holding on and then letting go, trotting beside me, cheering me on. I was the happiest boy in Newark when I got a bike for Christmas that year, and I've been riding ever since. That night stood out in my mind as a milestone I should have shared with my father, but I've always been grateful to Tony, not just for helping me to achieve something that seemed so important to me at the time, but also for the grown-up way that he dealt with my feelings. He didn't make fun of me or belittle me in that moment when I felt most vulnerable, and his generosity made me a bit less afraid to try new things and even to reach out for help.

I zeroed in on Tony's tired, leathery face as he sat on the aluminum gray bench adjacent to the emergency department. His eyes looked empty, his face unshaven, his hair matted, and I wondered: *What happened to the eager, fun-loving boy who was just as ambitious and smart as I was?*

One time as kids we came up with the brilliant idea of making homemade wine. We found old mayonnaise jars, filled them with grapes, water, and sugar, and then hid them in Tony's basement. I can't even remember what prompted our little experiment. We were no more than twelve years old; we had probably read the ingredients for wine somewhere and naïvely thought that was all it took. I can only imagine the bewilderment Tony's mother must have felt if she ever discovered those jars. I have no idea whether she ever actually did find them, but I was away in college when she suffered a stroke and died. His father died a few years later from complications related to long-term alcohol abuse.

As a kid, Tony swore he'd never be like his old man. When his father staggered into the house once after a day of drinking, Tony whispered to me, "I hate him!" The two of us also mocked the drug addicts who stumbled around the neighborhood, bug-eyed and begging. We just assumed we would do better. But something began to change around middle school. All of a sudden, it was no longer cool to raise our hands in class and call, "Pick me, pick me, oh, please pick me," vying for the teacher's attention. If you liked school, as I did, you pretended you couldn't stand it, like everybody else. If you got good grades, you hid them. And you'd just about die of embarrassment if you had to go up on stage to collect an award for academic achievement. The only kids who seemed proud of that kind of stuff were the geeky dudes who had no friends. Nobody ever showed us all the places that road could lead—at least nobody that mattered to us.

My friends and I were teenagers when we started experimenting with alcohol, sneaking a sip from our parents' bottles of Bacardi or pooling our money so somebody's big brother could buy us beer from the corner store. It seems silly now, but we all just wanted one another's approval. We wanted to seem cool, like the older guys around us. Tony soon started smoking marijuana; that was his cocktail. I always had an excuse for why I didn't want to do it. Truth be told, I had a feeling that if I started sliding down that hole, I'd keep falling deeper and deeper. I'd seen it happen to my sister Fellease, and to my older brother Kenny, who was an alcoholic. I was a freshman in college when a fight at a local bar left him paralyzed on his right side and confined to a wheelchair. Though he now lives in a home for the disabled, he hasn't had a drink in twenty years and is a happier, more peaceful person. My friend Tony had slid down that same dark hole. He dropped out of high school, married at eighteen, had more children than he could afford to raise (five was the last I'd heard), and got hooked on heroin. The drugs probably became his escape, his way of checking out so he wouldn't have to confront all of his broken dreams. Then he didn't have a clue how to begin piecing his life back together. He worked sporadically as a truck driver, but the deeper he got into drugs, the less he was able to hold down a steady job. The pull from the street was greater than his will or his ability to resist it.

Rick, the mutual friend who'd brought Tony to the hospital, explained that he had to leave to take care of some business, and I finally walked over to Tony, who was still sitting in the waiting room. How cool would it have been if he had become a doctor, too, and two old friends who'd once tried to make wine together in their basement as kids could laugh about it now and discuss the latest lifesaving procedure, or stand in the Fish Bowl and check out vacation sites on the computer? When he saw me, Tony stood. He did his best to appear cheerful, like in the old days when he wore a constant smile. We talked about how long it had been since we'd seen each other. Before long, Tony's eyes fell from mine toward the floor. He was clearly embarrassed. Standing before me in raggedy, oil-stained jeans, a dingy white T-shirt, and well-worn, dirty sneakers, he looked like the desperate, drug-addicted homeless man he had become.

"I need help," he said finally, still staring at the floor.

I remembered how gingerly he had handled my feelings all those years ago, and that was all I needed to hear. I refused to pry deeper.

"I'll find a place for you to go, man. I don't care how far we have to search. The nurse will get you something to eat. Don't worry. I'm going to take care of you."

"Thank you, Marshall," he whispered through dry, chapped lips.

If this wasn't rock bottom, I couldn't imagine what was. But there was still hope. Tony wasn't dead, like Snake. And he wasn't in jail, like so many other of our boys. He was willing to go to rehab, and I was determined to find someplace for him to go. The chance that I could possibly make such a difference in Tony's life gave me a huge adrenaline rush, though I knew well the first challenge I faced. After years of trying to help my sister and other family members, I knew that finding a good residential treatment center would be difficult. The fact that I was a doctor didn't change the reality that there just aren't many residential drug rehabilitation centers out there. The few willing to take a patient with no insurance, no job, and no other means to pay were in public hospitals, and like at Beth, crowding at any of those medical centers was sure to be an issue. According to the 2010 National Survey on Drug Use and Health, 23.1 million people ages twelve and older needed treatment for illicit drugs or alcohol use, but only 2.6 million were treated in a specialty facility. Of the 20.5 million who were classified as needing help but didn't receive it, just 1,024,000 reported that they personally felt they needed treatment. And of those roughly one million people, only 341,000 (33.3 percent) reported that they had made an effort to get treatment; the majority of them, 683,000 (66.7 percent), reported making no effort at all.

I dashed back to the Fish Bowl, waited for the phone to be free, and began calling hospitals that I knew offered drug rehabilitation. I must have called about ten of them, starting with those close to Beth Israel. Finally, I found an open bed at a hospital in New York City. I rushed out to share the news with Tony. He'd gotten lucky, I told him. He'd been given the hospital's only slot. This was his chance to start anew. He signed the transfer papers, and two hours later an ambulance arrived to take him to the hospital, located about twenty miles away. I stood in the ambulance bay and watched as my old friend was helped inside the vehicle. I felt purposeful and optimistic, even though I'd been through this experience enough with my own family members to know that my intervention didn't necessarily guarantee a happy ending. I would check on Tony in a week or so, I thought, and maybe even take a trip to New York to offer support.

But the following week, Tony was back at Beth. It was impossible not to notice him as he wandered around outside the hospital.

He saw me speaking to a co-worker in the hall of the emergency department and knocked on the ambulance bay entry door. My spirits dropped at his once-again scruffy appearance, but he wore a giant smile. When I opened the door, I saw that he was holding two enormous chocolate bars in his left hand. He extended the other hand and thanked me for all that I had done. Then he immediately began explaining. He'd been admitted to the hospital the night I wrote the order, he said, but he was discharged the next day because he didn't have his Social Security card. Puzzled, I looked at him as if to say, *C'mon, dude, stop lying!*

He swore it was the truth. One thing I've learned about drug addicts is that a lie can fly out of their mouths with such ease that it sometimes feels like the truth to them.

"I swear to you, Marshall, they said it was impossible to bill me for my stay if they didn't have my information," Tony said, obviously having noticed the disappointment on my face. "They told me to come back to New Jersey and secure the proper paperwork and then they could help me." He paused. "Well, regardless, I have been clean for one week."

"Where are you staying now?" I asked.

Tony hesitated again. "I'm in a shelter in downtown Newark. It's cool. I have to be out by nine and back in by six."

Tony lifted his hand with the candy bars. "Say, why don't you take this candy off me for three dollars. Man, I'm hungry and could use the money to get something to eat."

I smiled in disbelief. I'd been a target the instant Tony saw me through the glass doors. He was hustling me, most likely to get high. Drug addicts are the best salesmen in the world. They can sell hot water on a summer day. I fumbled around in my pocket and came up with two dollars.

"Here, go get something to eat," I said, handing him the cash.

He pushed the chocolate bars my way. "Here you go."

"Naw, man, I'm all right," I said. "I can't eat that stuff. It tears my stomach up. Why don't you eat them? You said you were hungry."

He nodded. I felt like the basketball player who hustles to the sidelines in the last minutes of a close game, pulls back a stray ball headed out of bounds, gets it into the hands of the star player under the net, only to watch him stand there, refusing to go for the layup. A mix of anger, sadness, and disappointment rose inside me. I wanted to yell at Tony, make him see that the ball was in his hands, that he was just one leap from victory.

"Tony, you have got to get your life together," I said, exasperated. "You have a family, especially your children at home."

"I know, man. You're right. You'll see. I'm gonna straighten up. I'm done with getting high."

I couldn't say another word. My spirit was crushed—and maybe a bit of my ego, too. I'd wanted Tony to win this time, and I'd wanted to be the game changer. But to make a difference here, I'd need to put in a lot more effort, I realized, and I'd need a lot more patience. Anywhere from half to 90 percent of people with an addictive disease experience a relapse, statistics show. For alcohol and drug addiction, relapse often is chronic, especially with men, who are less inclined to participate in group counseling and therapy.

"Well, thanks again, man," Tony said, scurrying away. "I have to run, got to hustle up another dollar to get something to eat."

And with that, my old friend disappeared around the corner.

Where Can Family Members Go for Information on Treatment Options?*

Trying to locate appropriate treatment for a loved one, especially a program tailored to an individual's particular needs, can be a difficult process. However, there are some resources currently available to help with this process, including:

- The Substance Abuse and Mental Health Services Administration (SAMHSA) maintains a website (www.findtreatment.samhsa.gov) that shows the location of residential, outpatient, and hospital inpatient treatment programs for drug addiction and alcoholism throughout the country. This information is also accessible by calling 1-800-662-HELP.

- The National Suicide Prevention Lifeline (1-800-273-TALK) offers more than just suicide prevention—it can also help with a host of issues, including drug and alcohol abuse, and can connect individuals with a nearby professional.

- The National Alliance on Mental Illness (www.nami.org) and Mental Health America (www.mentalhealthamerica.net) are alliances of non-profit, self-help support organizations for patients and families dealing with a variety of mental disorders. Both have state and local affiliates throughout the country and may be especially helpful for patients with co-morbid conditions.

- The American Academy of Addiction Psychiatry and the American Academy of Child and Adolescent Psychiatry each have physician locator tools posted on their websites at www.aaap.org and www.aacap.org, respectively.

- For information about participating in a clinical trial testing promising substance abuse interventions, contact NIDA's National Drug Abuse Treatment Clinical Trials Network at www.drugabuse.gov/ctn/, or visit NIH's website at www.clinicaltrials.gov.

*Excerpt from *Principles of Drug Addiction Treatment: A Research-Based Guide* (Second Edition), sponsored by the National Institutes of Health's National Institute on Drug Abuse

10

RUSSIAN ROULETTE

My old friend Tony's eyes provided the first clue that he was depressed. They looked empty, and everything about him that day at the hospital said that he had lost hope. I suspect that when he first began feeling that way, he turned to alcohol and drugs to dull the pain, instead of seeking help for depression. Practically every day I see signs of untreated depression in the faces and behaviors of men and women I encounter on the street and in the emergency department. The hollow eyes are a familiar telltale sign. It's as if you can see through them into empty souls. Many of those who suffer, especially in minority communities, don't see depression as a medical condition that is as treatable as high blood pressure. More times than not, they refuse to seek help because they fear being labeled "crazy." If they are religious, they sometimes see their persistent depression as an indication of poor faith, which only deepens their despair.

According to a major 2007 psychiatric study financed by the National Institute of Mental Health, black Americans, including those of Caribbean descent, are less likely than white Americans to suffer from major depressive disorders, but the struggles of black Americans with depression tend to be more chronic and more severe. The National Survey of American Life included one of the largest populations of black participants for a study of its type—3,570 African Americans, 1,621 blacks of Caribbean descent who immigrated to the United States or were born there, and 891 non-Hispanic whites ages eighteen and older. It showed that fewer than half of African Americans and just one-quarter of black Caribbeans with major depression undergo treatment. Untreated depression is the leading cause of suicide. Various studies have shown that African Americans and Latinos are the least likely of all racial groups to commit suicide. But sometimes they remain locked in their private hell—until their sadness turns to desperation.

Throughout my residency, I treated many patients who wound up in the emergency department after swallowing too many pills on purpose. Once, I even pronounced a newly divorced man in his sixties dead: He had draped an American flag across his body, plunged a butcher knife through his chest, and bled to death before he made it to the emergency room. But nothing prepared me for Juan, a twenty-four-year-old from Puerto Rico who landed in the emergency department during one of my shifts about a year after shooting himself in the head.

He had survived the suicide attempt, but the gunshot had left him blind and disfigured. His eyes had been removed during emergency surgery after the shooting, and he had not yet healed enough for prosthetics. The sockets were infected and leaking pus, which is why his parents had brought him to the hospital that day. Juan was a big guy, about six feet tall, 230 pounds, with short black hair. A scar on both sides of his face, just underneath his temples, indicated the path of the bullet. He towered over both of his parents, a plainly dressed couple in their late forties or early fifties. They seemed distraught and weary as I motioned for them to step into the hallway with me to talk. A translator provided by the hospital followed them out of the room. The father, a medium-built man with black hair and graying temples, stood off to the side, stoic and silent. The mother's salt-and-pepper hair hung straight, just past her shoulders, with the sides tucked behind her ears. She wore no makeup, and her face bore the permanent etchings of worry. The weight of her guilt was palpable. She turned to the translator and spoke in rapid-fire Spanish. She wanted her son checked for depression. She clearly blamed herself and was taking no chances that Juan might hurt himself again. I looked down at his chart, which noted that he'd been seen a few times in the psychiatric unit of the emergency department in the months since the shooting. I assured Mrs. Ortiz that I would make sure Juan saw the psychiatrist when I was done.

I had already begun to piece together the story from the medical records and the scars on Juan's face, but I wanted to know more. "What happened?" I asked as sensitively as I could.

She covered her face with her hands, shaking her head as though she still could not believe it. And all of her pain came flowing out.

He had been a beautiful, happy boy, she said. They had come to America when he was just a baby, to give him a better life. They'd settled in Perth Amboy, New Jersey, between Newark and New Brunswick, and worked long and hard to provide for him. But something went wrong in his teen years. He shut them out, started staying out late, and sometimes locked himself in his bedroom for hours. His temper was explosive; a simple request for him to take out the trash or clean his room would send him into a rage. Other times, he was sullen and sad. Maybe it was just some weird teenage phase, the parents thought. Maybe he'd grow out of it soon, and they'd get their happy, energetic boy back.

But time didn't improve Juan's condition. He dropped out of high school, couldn't keep a steady job, and could never earn enough from odd jobs to leave his parents' house. He never brought his friends over. Then one evening, when his mother made it home from work, the house seemed quieter than usual. There was no loud rap music coming from Juan's room—in fact, she didn't hear him stirring at all. After a while, she took the chance of making him angry and knocked on his door. When he didn't answer, she pushed it open slightly, peeked inside, and there he was, sprawled in the middle of the floor in a pool of his own blood. A gun lay next to his hand. She screamed and dropped to her knees, begging and praying. She crawled to the nightstand, yanked down the telephone, and punched in 911. She screamed to the dispatcher in her broken English: "Help! My son been shot!"

My heart ached for this family. As the mother stood there, trembling, weeping, recalling that awful night, her husband eased to her side and slipped his arm around her waist.

"It's not your fault, Mrs. Ortiz," I said, trying to reassure her. "You did the best you could for him. And you did the right thing to bring him to the hospital today."

I explained that Juan had developed an eye socket infection, and I described how to administer the antibiotic ointment that I was prescribing. I also prescribed antibiotic pills and wished them well. But I will never forget the disturbing image of Juan, a once strong young man, now blind and disfigured by his own hand. According to the National Institute of Mental Health, there are eleven suicide attempts for every death. Juan probably had no idea that there was a healthy way out of the darkness that had driven him to such desperation. And even though his parents saw him changing, they knew nothing about depression and where it could lead. Neither did I, the last time I saw my childhood friend Lil' Moe.

He was my basketball buddy. As kids, the two of us shot hoops together under the blazing sun almost every day. I was in awe of his crossover dribble and pull-up jump shot—*swoosh,* it was all net. His nickname at first was Showtime because he was so entertaining to watch. He was the tallest kid in the second grade, but the rest of us quickly caught up, and by the time we reached sixth grade, he was the shortest. His interests switched to boxing, and his older brother, who was known around the neighborhood as Big Moe, became his trainer. When it seemed my friend would become his big brother's protégé, everybody began calling the little brother Lil' Moe. I went with him to the gym a few times, and once or twice even sparred with him, but it didn't take me long to figure out that boxing just wasn't for me. It didn't make much sense to me to allow someone to beat me upside my head and body. But Lil' Moe excelled and quickly gained respect for his fast hands and knockout power. He had extreme talent and ambition and a burning desire to master everything that was presented to him as a challenge. He was also a fun-loving, down-to-earth guy whom everyone loved. He soon became the local junior glove champion. Word quickly spread on the street not to go up against Lil' Moe, and his street credentials grew exponentially after an encounter at the neighborhood skating rink one night with a much-feared neighborhood bully named Rock.

Rock was from the Dayton Street projects, and he'd roam the neighborhood, pick a target, and demand everything from money to clothes and jewelry. Everybody was scared of Rock. I remember looking out my bedroom window once and seeing him handle another guy on the street. They were fighting, and Rock had pulled his own shirt off. Rock's opponent was six, maybe eight inches taller, but true to form, Rock connected on several punches and kicks, knocking the guy out right there on the street, for all to see. Rock trained in boxing as well as martial arts, but to reinforce his domination, he also carried a gun. He'd occasionally pull it out during a confrontation to make sure everybody knew the deal. Some guys even paid him for protection.

The funny thing is, Rock was a little dude. He stood no taller than five feet seven inches and was outweighed by practically everyone he encountered in the ring and on the street. But he could fight; he knocked his opponents out. And, of course, he always had that gun. Everybody in the neighborhood measured their own street credibility by Rock's. If you were a part of his camp, you never had to worry about anyone else targeting or testing you. Rock had a virtual army, with generals and soldiers ready to take on any task.

Lil' Moe was never on Rock's hit list, in part because Rock and Lil' Moe's brother, Big Moe, had once been best friends. They'd trained together at a local community center. But as they got older, they went their separate ways. Big Moe was the opposite of Rock. For every bad thing Rock did, it seemed Big Moe did something positive. He didn't do drugs, and he volunteered his time at the community center. He was the one who got his little brother involved in boxing.

Lil' Moe and I had to be at least five years younger than Rock, which felt at the time like a different generation. We weren't considered a threat to him or his empire. Actually, we were excited if Rock spoke to us or knew our names as he prowled through the neighborhood. He would walk past us as we played and at times acknowledge us by shooting the ball during a basketball game. He would shoot a few jumpers and keep moving. This only increased his popularity among the guys my age and left us feeling important.

"Rock shot some hoops with me today," I'd say, bragging to friends who hadn't been there, and I could see the envy in my boys' eyes. Even the teachers at my grammar school who didn't live in the neighborhood were familiar with the character named Rock.

"Who *is* this Rock?" they'd ask after hearing his name again and again.

Nobody could have guessed that a new neighborhood king was about to be crowned that breezy spring night as we talked about the fun we'd have later at the skating rink. It was Friday, and soon everybody would be heading there. It was a neighborhood tradition. By the time the rain came pouring down, we were all circling the rink with top-twenty hits blasting and colorful lights flashing. Lil' Moe was gliding with such rhythm across the waxed hardwood floors that he appeared to be floating. He made a nice twisting move, and just then, a girl tripped and fell right in front of him. He swerved to avoid running over her, but he went flying directly into Rock. The impact lifted Rock into the air, and he hit the ground with a loud thud. Embarrassed and furious, Rock hopped up and tore into Lil' Moe. And just like that, the fight was on, skates and all.

It lasted for what seemed like an eternity, and to everyone's shock, Lil' Moe got the best of Rock. With both of them wobbling on skates, Lil' Moe dodged all of Rock's best moves, while throwing his own combination of punches, leaving Rock's face and his pride bloodied. For weeks afterward, the neighborhood seemed to collectively hold our breath, waiting for the sad moment when Rock would exact his revenge. To our astonishment, that day never came. Everyone suspected Big Moe had negotiated peace. But Lil' Moe became the new neighborhood hero for putting Rock in his place.

Eventually, I went away to college and lost touch with Lil' Moe, who stayed behind in the neighborhood. When I returned to Newark to start my residency at Beth, I ran into him outside his old building in the neighborhood. It was during the Thanksgiving holidays, and he was working as a stock clerk at the local grocery store. I could tell that dark days were upon him. He had those hollow eyes, was overweight, and was missing more than half his teeth. He appeared disheveled. To overcome the uncomfortable silence, I asked if he was still boxing, but I immediately felt ashamed for doing so. He looked at me with a bit of confusion, as if I should have known by looking at him that it was a crazy question.

"Man, I haven't picked up the gloves in years," he mumbled.

He told me that life had dealt him some serious challenges: His mother had died, Big Moe had been seriously injured in a car accident, and Lil' Moe's girlfriend had just left him for another dude. "And I'm stuck here," he said. He told me he'd heard about my going off to college, and he talked about his own regrets.

"Man, my life would have been totally different if I'd stayed in school."

I could tell he was depressed, but I was at a loss for the best way to reach out to him. "Man, I work right at Beth Israel," I told him. "If you ever want to come by, just give me a call."

In retrospect, I realize that I must have come across as distant, disconnected, and maybe even disingenuous. If I could have peeked into the future, I might have really tried to connect, to remind Lil' Moe who he was, and let him know that there was help available. Instead, I simply shook Lil' Moe's hand and promised to stay in touch. I'm sure we both thought we'd see each other again. There's always tomorrow, right?

That was 1999. I didn't hear his name again until a few years later, when a co-worker in the emergency department asked one day if I'd heard about what happened to Lil' Moe. I hadn't, but I knew intuitively as my co-worker launched into the story that it wouldn't be good news.

It was New Year's Eve, and Lil' Moe got together with a few friends from the neighborhood to celebrate. They were smoking, drinking, and playing cards, when Lil' Moe, probably already loaded, pulled out a gun and tried to recruit players for a game of Russian roulette. No one was willing. He called them cowards, but still none of them budged. The crazy thing is, no one tried to talk him out of it either. Perhaps they were all too drunk to realize he was serious. Even when he put the gun to his head and pulled the trigger, they figured he was just fooling around. Surely, he'd taken out all the bullets. Who would be foolish enough to play this crazy game with a real bullet in the barrel? He fired three times, they said—*click, click, click*—before *BOOM!* Next thing his friends knew, twenty-six-year-old Lil' Moe was down, and his brains were splattered across the wall.

Major panic followed—the screams, the frantic call to 911, the flashing red lights, and the body bag. Then came the regrets. His friends were full of them. They wished they'd paid more attention, insisted he get help. They wished they'd halted his ridiculous suicide mission. They wished they'd stepped in when they still had a chance.

But just like that, Lil' Moe's tomorrow—and his friends' chances to step in—had vanished.

The Warning Signs for Suicide*

The following signs may mean someone is at risk for suicide. The risk is greater if a behavior is new or has increased and if it seems related to a painful event, loss, or change. Seek help as soon as possible by contacting a mental health professional or by calling the Lifeline at **1-800-273-TALK (8255)** if you or someone you know is:

- Talking about wanting to die or to kill oneself
- Looking for a way to kill oneself, such as searching online or buying a gun
- Talking about feeling hopeless or having no reason to live
- Talking about feeling trapped or in unbearable pain
- Talking about being a burden to others
- Increasing the use of alcohol or drugs
- Acting anxious or agitated; behaving recklessly
- Sleeping too little or too much
- Withdrawing or feeling isolated
- Showing rage or talking about seeking revenge
- Displaying extreme mood swings

HOW TO BE HELPFUL TO SOMEONE WHO IS THREATENING SUICIDE*

- Be direct. Talk openly and matter-of-factly about suicide.
- Be willing to listen. Allow expressions of feelings. Accept the feelings.
- Be non-judgmental. Don't debate whether suicide is right or wrong, or whether feelings are good or bad. Don't lecture on the value of life.
- Get involved. Become available. Show interest and support.
- Don't dare him or her to do it.
- Don't act shocked. This will put distance between you.
- Don't be sworn to secrecy. Seek support.

- Offer hope that alternatives are available but do not offer glib reassurance.
- Take action. Remove means, such as guns or stockpiled pills.
- Get help from persons or agencies specializing in crisis intervention and suicide prevention.

Reprinted from the National Suicide Prevention Lifeline

11

NO AIR

The patient's face was a blur as the stretcher whizzed past me in the halls of Beth Israel one summer afternoon in 2002. But I recognized his dreads. Those thick, shoulder-length locks told me what my pager alert moments earlier could not: that I knew this patient.

I ran to catch up. My eyes followed his oversized white T-shirt to his face, confirming his identity. It was my friend Mark, the cook and cashier in the hospital's ancillary cafeteria. He'd suffered a severe asthma attack.

"I'm here, man," I said, trotting beside the stretcher as emergency workers rolled it to the resuscitation room.

I had warned Mark about the cigarettes. Smoking and asthma are a deadly combination, and Mark knew it. But, like Mr. Tate and the millions of people in the country addicted to smoking, Mark wouldn't—or couldn't—quit. He probably thought he had forever to change. He surely couldn't have guessed that forever would come so suddenly, on this beautiful summer day as he sat on the passenger side of his best friend's car, idling at a traffic light, just moments from his destination. When the EMS team arrived, Mark was barely breathing. His six-foot frame lay stretched out on the pavement, as still as the air. His best friend, Shawn, kneeled beside him and held him. Emergency workers quickly inserted a breathing tube, administered intravenous drugs, and rushed him to Beth, where my team worked frantically to save his life. But the cardiac monitor showed no pulse, no heartbeat. I looked down at my friend's lifeless body and knew it would take more than my medical skill and strong will to bring him back. It would take a miracle.

Mark was one of the friendliest, most upbeat dudes I'd ever met. Most days, I'd rush into the cafeteria just before my shift or during a break, and he'd be there behind the counter, with his condiment-stained apron shielding his stylish clothes. Just a few months older than me, he was the cook, cashier, delivery guy, everyman, doing whatever it took to keep the small operation running smoothly. The main cafeteria on the second floor was closed part of the day, so the smaller one was always bustling with hospital workers who watched the clock while trying to grab a quick bite or a cup of caffeine, and family members needing food or respite from sick loved ones. But no matter how busy he was, Mark never failed to acknowledge me. It really touched me how much my presence at Beth Israel seemed to mean to many of the hospital's hourly workers, many of whom had grown up in Newark. Beth hired heavily from the surrounding neighborhoods, and when I joined the staff, word circulated quickly that the new young black doctor had grown up in the hood, not far from the hospital.

"Proud of you, man," I heard again and again from the orderlies, janitors, cooks, and clerks, who became my first friends. Thanks to people like Mark, I loved coming to work. Mark went out of his way to be kind. He'd spot me in line and flash his brilliant smile, thirty-two perfectly aligned teeth set against flawless mahogany skin. "Hey, Doc, I got your drink ready to go," he'd say, reaching over the counter to hand me my regular, a large hazelnut coffee with cream and two sugars.

We became friends one day when I was picking up my regular.

Traffic was relatively light in the cafeteria that day, and Mark joined me on my side of the counter. He carried a pack of cigarettes, and I assumed he was headed outside for a break.

"Doc, you leaving?" he asked.

"Yeah, I got to make it upstairs," I said. "I heard things are already pretty busy today."

We headed toward the exit, and I held the door open for Mark and followed him into the hallway, just short of the escalator. It was a Friday, and only a few hours stood between Mark and his days off. But his spirits seemed unusually heavy. And I could tell he wanted to talk.

"I wanted to be a doctor once," he began matter-of-factly. "But I messed up in school. Following the wrong crowd, you know, and then dropped out." He paused and shook his head, reflecting on the past. "I had a bunch of toos. Too fast, too grown, and too dumb for my own good. Look at me now. I'm working in this dead-end job, no future in sight."

It surprised me to see Mark in such a mood. He continued without any prompting, "Man, the only good thing that ever happened to me was my baby girl. You've probably seen her around here. I was eighteen when she was born. I was so happy, though if I had to do it all over again, I'd wait. I got a job as soon as I found out my girl was pregnant. I figured I would work double shifts, sixteen hours a day, whatever it took to give her and my baby a better life. You know, I didn't want her coming up like me, without her daddy. I promised her and her mother when she was born, right there in the delivery room, that I would always be there for them. The years went by and, you know, I never made it back to high school, let alone college. Before you know it, you're working hard just to stay in place."

By then Mark was fidgeting with his cigarettes. The nicotine was calling, and I knew he had only a few minutes for break. The emergency department wouldn't shut down if I got there a few minutes late, I figured. I motioned for him to follow me outside. As soon as we stepped onto the concrete, he reached for his lighter, pulled out a cigarette, and touched it to the flame.

"I know what you mean," I said. "It's so hard to get ahead. But it's never too late to go after your dreams."

He took a long drag on the cigarette. "I've been here at Beth ten years. I do it all, man, but I'll never own this café. I'm just a worker to the owner, nothing else. I'm reminded every day that I have to take shit from people. They walk all over you when they know they can. But what can I do? Just walk away?" He chuckled. "That's why I'm so proud of you, Doc. You did it, man."

Mark's story moved and humbled me. I knew the frustration of feeling trapped by your circumstances. But I'd also seen firsthand that the seemingly impossible can become possible with determination and hard work. Talking to Mark that day helped me realize more than ever that my success was not just about me. I was living the dream of so many others who had found their own dreams smacked down by life: the black cooks, orderlies, and janitors who joked with me in the halls; the elderly men and women in the community who went out of their way to wish me well; and even the tough guys who locked me into their gaze as they lay dying.

Mark finished his cigarette, stamped out the butt, and then reached into his pocket. I was stunned by what he pulled out: an albuterol inhaler. Until that moment, I had no idea he had asthma. He quickly took two puffs from the small pump and returned it to his pocket.

"Now, you know better, Mark. Asthma and smoking—come on, man," I said in my best cool doctor approach. I wanted him to know that I didn't approve, but I also didn't want to alienate him by being too preachy.

"I know, Doc, I know," Mark said. "I shouldn't be smoking."

We made our way back into the hospital and headed our separate ways. Every time I saw him after that, we chatted about sports, music, the news of the day, or his eleven-year-old daughter, Trina. Soon after I met him, I was passing through the cafeteria and saw a cute little girl sitting behind the cash register, and Mark introduced me to her. Trina had the same rich brown complexion as her dad, a dimpled smile, and hair that flowed over her shoulders in small, neat braids with colorful rubber bands on the tips. I soon discovered that she came to the hospital nearly every day after school and sat at the register with an air of pride and confidence. No one could tell her that the small cafeteria wasn't her daddy's place. While waiting for him to get off work and take her home, she dutifully did her homework. She beamed in his presence and glanced at him for approval when she spoke.

A couple of times, I ran into Mark in the emergency department, where he'd come to get a breathing treatment when his asthma got out of control. About a quarter of all people who visit the emergency rooms throughout the country are there due to symptoms related to asthma. The number of those who suffer from it—an estimated 20 million Americans (one in fifteen people)—has been growing steadily across all racial and ethnic groups since the early 1980s. But the condition is slightly more prevalent and much more severe among African Americans, who are three times more likely to be hospitalized because of it. That seemed evident to me early in my tenure at Beth by the large number of black patients filling the recliners lined against a wall, there exclusively for those receiving nebulizer breathing treatments. The nebulizer converts liquid medication into a mist that can be easily inhaled through a mask and quickly absorbed by the lungs to open constricted airways.

"Doc, when you are having an asthma attack, it really is like breathing through a straw," Mark once explained during a brief chat. "Can you imagine that? You are exhausted, using all your muscles and energy just to get a small amount of air. Feels like you're being buried alive."

Mark had been diagnosed with asthma as a child and had been hospitalized for it several times through the years, but he'd learned to accept and manage his condition, he told me. He knew the triggers: some pets, carpets, heat, certain medicines, exercise, and, especially, smoke. But he just figured that with his inhaler, he was in control. Still, I reminded him every chance I got: "You know, cigarettes aren't helping the matter."

As usual, he would promise to quit: "Next year, Doc. I promise."

The last time I asked if he'd quit smoking he told me he was down to eight cigarettes a day. "That's better than the two packs a day I used to smoke," he added.

Mark was flirting with death, though I'm sure he didn't see it that way. But one in five deaths each year is attributed to cigarette smoking. More people die from smoking than from HIV, illegal drug use, alcohol use, motor vehicle injuries, suicide, and murders combined.

For an asthmatic, smoking causes irritation of the airways, greatly enhancing the chances of an attack, and African American asthma patients are three times more likely than their white counterparts to die during an attack. Most of these deaths could be avoided, though, with proper treatment and preventative measures.

The same is true with many other medical conditions, yet every day I treat patients who keep smoking despite a diagnosis of asthma or emphysema, or keep eating high-fat or salt- and sugar-laden foods despite their diabetes, hypertension, or heart condition or the threat of developing them. And even after diagnosis, they are inconsistent with their medications, either neglecting to take them as prescribed or skipping them altogether. These destructive patterns seem more acute in poor urban communities, where people frequently use cigarettes, drugs, and food to cope with stress and the miserable circumstances that often come with poverty. And the truth is perhaps easy to ignore for long periods of time because the human body is resilient and can withstand much abuse—until it can't.

The day an ambulance carried him to Beth Israel, Mark had hopped into Shawn's car for a quick trip across town to visit another friend. Sometimes, when I think of Mark and what happened that day, I imagine him flashing that easy, ever-present smile, showing every one of his flawless teeth, low-riding on the passenger side of Shawn's Mazda RX-7. I can see the two friends, bouncing to the rap beat thumping from the stereo as the car rolled through the streets of Newark. I can almost feel the hot, humid air rushing through the open window, causing Mark's shoulder-length dreads to flap in the wind. I can smell the cigarette burning between his mahogany fingers.

If only Mark could have that moment back . . .

He was wheezing when he sat straight up in the car and began fishing furiously through his pants pockets. He pulled out his albuterol inhaler, wrapped his lips around the mouthpiece, and squeezed the pump with his fingers. A tiny bit of mist came out. He squeezed again, and again. The canister was empty.

Hearing his friend's wheezing grow louder, Shawn panicked and sped through the light. I can only guess that he figured paramedics could get to them faster than he could drive to the hospital, and so he raced the one block to their friend John's house, and within seconds was whipping the car into the driveway. As soon as the car stopped, Mark hopped out and began jumping up and down and slapping his chest, as if to force the air into his lungs. Shawn punched 911 into his cell phone, honked repeatedly, and jumped out of the car just as Mark collapsed onto the pavement. It all happened so quickly. John and his parents rushed outside and became hysterical, then ran back inside to grab the telephone to call Mark's family. Neighbors and passersby gathered and watched helplessly. Paramedics arrived within minutes and quickly loaded Mark into the ambulance.

At the hospital, Shawn seemed in shock, recounting every detail of the story, as if to convince himself he'd done all he could do to save his boy. But guilt was eating away at him. "I shouldn't have given him that cigarette," he said, blaming himself.

Mark had asked for the cigarette, and he'd promised Shawn— just as he'd promised me many times—that he was going to quit smoking. I was angry at myself for not pushing Mark harder to stop, and I was angry at him for gambling with his life every time he took a puff. This time, he'd lost it all. There would be no miracle. At just twenty-nine years old, Mark was dead. He had died before he made it to the hospital, and my medical team could not bring him back.

Shortly after I made the official pronouncement, Mark's girlfriend and daughter joined other family members in a small private room at the hospital. They were all in shock, hugging and consoling one another. I introduced myself to them and expressed my condolences. Trina recognized me from the times I'd joked with her in the cafeteria. Her mother was weeping when she led the child over to me and asked me to tell her—she couldn't do it. I'd broken bad news to families many times before, but never like this. I knew this little girl. I knew how much she adored her father and how hard he had worked to make life better for her. I started there.

"Your daddy loved you so much," I said, handing Trina an apple juice. "You remember how he sometimes had asthma attacks and couldn't catch his breath? Well, this time, he had a really bad one. We did everything we could to save him, but I'm sorry to say that we couldn't."

Trina certainly must have known something was seriously wrong from the grieving all around her, but she didn't want to hear it. "Stop saying that, Dr. Davis," she replied. "My daddy is downstairs."

She knew better. She didn't take her eyes off me, and the seriousness of my face confirmed what she didn't want to believe. She suddenly began to sob.

A few days later, I attended Mark's wake. Perry's Funeral Home in Newark was packed with flowers and mourners, including many familiar faces from Beth Israel. I sat in the back, full of sadness, looking at a large portrait of Mark sitting on an easel next to his oak coffin. The image in that picture was the one I would carry in my memory: Mark in his oversized white T-shirt, long dreads, and that wide, perfect smile.

My caffeine runs at the hospital were never quite the same after that. I missed my friend, and every time I walked into his old spot, I couldn't help thinking: another young brother, gone too soon.

Things People With Asthma Can Do to Manage It:

- Have an individual management plan (a written action plan developed with your doctor) containing:
    - Your medications (controller and quick relief)
    - Your asthma triggers (the environmental or other factors that cause your attack)
    - What to do when you have an attack
- Educate yourself and others about how to reduce your risk of an attack:
    - Reducing your exposure to house dust mites
        - Use bedding encasement
        - Wash bed linens weekly
        - Avoid down fillings
        - Limit stuffed animals to those that can be washed
    - Reducing humidity level (between 30 percent and 50 percent EPR-3)
    - Reducing exposure to environmental tobacco smoke
    - Reducing exposure to cockroaches
        - Remove as many standing water and food sources as possible to avoid cockroaches
    - Reducing exposure to pets
        - People who are allergic should not allow them in the home
        - At a minimum, pets should not be allowed in the bedroom of someone who is allergic
    - Reducing exposure to mold
        - Eliminating mold and moist conditions that permit mold
- Seek help from asthma resources:
    - Centers for Disease Control and Prevention (www.cdc.gov/asthma/faqs.htm)
    - Allergy and Asthma Network, Mothers of Asthmatics (www.aanma.org/)

- American Academy of Allergy, Asthma and Immunology (www.aaaai.org/home.aspx)
- American Academy of Family Physicians (familydoctor.org/familydoctor/en/diseases-conditions/asthma/treatment/asthma-action-plan.html)
- American Academy of Pediatrics (www.aap.org/healthtopics/asthma.cfm)
- Asthma and Allergy Foundation of America (www.aafa.org/)
- The National Environmental Education Foundation (www.neefusa.org/health/asthma/index.htm)
- Join an asthma support group

Source: Centers for Disease Control and Prevention

12

KILLING US SOFTLY

My name crackled through the walkie-talkie, rising above the usual clatter in the emergency department one afternoon in late summer of 2002. I rushed across the room and grabbed the unit from the counter: "Dr. Davis here, go ahead."

By then I was the doctor in charge. Just weeks earlier, I had become an "attending" physician, one of the doctors responsible for supervising residents. It had happened overnight. On June 30, 2002, I was a resident myself; then, at midnight, three years to the minute after my residency had started, it was over. Not only was I now on my own to make decisions about patient care, I was also in charge of others. Residents are allowed to assess and treat patients, but the treatment plans must be pre-approved by the attending physician, who closely monitors the young doctors. Since Beth is a teaching hospital, after the third year every resident who stays moves into the role of an attending physician, working as an instructor and passing on the details of emergency medicine to the next class of residents and interns. Other residents move on to work in smaller community-based hospitals, without the added responsibility of teaching.

"We have a seven-hundred-pound female coming to your hospital," the emergency technician said through the walkie-talkie.

"Can you please have a stretcher set up outside and someone to lend a hand with her? We're five minutes out."

A seven-hundred-pound patient would require major improvisation to our usual lifesaving procedures. I motioned for every available member of my team to head to the ambulance bay.

"Is she stable?" I asked. "What are her vital signs?"

The technician paused for a second. "She currently has labored breathing and an extremely faint pulse. The medic is starting a line, and we're doing our best to secure her airway."

I yelled out to the nurse in charge to get everything in place for the incoming patient, and then headed for the door. Within minutes, siren blaring, red lights flashing, the ambulance was backing into the bay area. When the back doors of the ambulance swung open, I was stunned. I'd never seen a human being this size before. The patient's body spilled over the sides of the gurney, leaving no grabbing room to maneuver the stretcher from the ambulance. It took all ten members of my emergency team, including me, to transfer her to the oversized bed that we had wheeled outside. Sweat poured from our foreheads as we strained to lift her. Every one of us concentrated intensely to avoid dropping our patient, an African American woman, whose face looked young, like she was in her late thirties or early forties. Her ankles were the size of my thighs, and her toenails were unusually long and dark. She had silky salt-and-pepper hair, which had been braided neatly into two shoulder-length plaits. I focused on keeping her upper body as upright as possible and her airway open.

The transfer from the ambulance went smoothly, considering, but we were losing time. Every step that we normally zipped through with ease was much slower than usual—time away from treating our patient. The emergency team rolled the bed as quickly as we could from the parking lot to the resuscitation bay. On the way, the medic filled me in on what he knew. The patient's name was Gloria, and the call for help had come from her neighbor, who checked in on her periodically. Gloria had been living alone for the past six months and was mostly bedridden because walking had become too painful. She had told her approximate weight to her neighbor, who had wanted to call for help sooner. But Gloria had begged her not to alert anyone. On the morning of the crisis, however, the neighbor had let herself in to check on Gloria and found her struggling to breathe and complaining of pressure in her chest. When the paramedics arrived, Gloria was barely conscious, lying in her own feces on a urine-soaked mattress in her bedroom. Snacks and empty junk food containers littered the room. Empty plates coated with dried food were scattered on the floor beside the bed. The stench in the room was almost intolerable, they said.

Gloria moaned as we began to work on her. Finally, we managed to get a stronger pulse. I stretched an extra-large cuff around her upper arm, but it wouldn't fit. I slid it down to her forearm and took her blood pressure there; it was extremely low. An EKG showed a bumpy, abnormal heart rhythm. It wasn't possible to do a CAT scan to determine whether she'd had a stroke. The maximum weight our machine could handle was 350 pounds. In non-emergency situations, we sent heavier patients to be scanned at the local zoo.

The paramedics had managed to insert an IV in her hand, but it was barely functioning and insufficient for all that we needed to do. We had to place a central line that would give us direct access to a large vein, where we could deliver fluids and, if necessary, lifesaving medication. In ordinary circumstances, we would have had three options: the jugular vein in the neck, the subclavian in the chest, or the femoral in the groin. Gloria had practically no neck, so going for the jugular was out of the question. The risks of the subclavian procedure were too high: The subclavian vein was too close to the lungs, and I didn't want to risk the potential deadly consequences from puncturing the wrong thing. There was no way she would survive a collapsed lung. Plus, there would be no time for an X-ray to assure that the line was in the right place. I had to try for the femoral vein in her groin area. I called out for help, and two nurses rushed to my side. They pushed up the mound of abdominal fat hanging down over Gloria's lap. Nurses and doctors are accustomed to seeing unimaginable things and are not easily grossed out, but all of us winced when we saw the abundance of raw sores and pockets of fungus growing within the folds of Gloria's skin. The smell was putrid, like rotting meat.

I swabbed the area quickly with Betadine and draped a sterile paper cloth over it. My gloved fingers searched for the slight pulse of the artery closest to the vein. After several tries, I felt a faint throb, and inserted a large needle right next to it into the femoral vein. A flash of dark red blood into the syringe told me I'd found the right spot. I continued the procedure, but just as I was about done, things got worse. Gloria's body suddenly became still and unresponsive. The cardiac monitor flatlined. I quickly checked her femoral artery for a pulse. Nothing. She was in cardiac arrest. My team immediately began CPR, but that process was hampered, too, by the circumstances. In most cases, we slipped a board between the patient and the thin mattress of the stretcher, keeping the body stiff and allowing the heart to absorb the weight of the chest compressions. But the oversized bed where Gloria lay—the only bed that could accommodate her size—had a regular soft mattress. We couldn't put the board under her because it was too small. Gloria sank into the mattress with every chest compression, which did little to jump-start her heart.

"Come on, Gloria," I whispered in frustration, as if she could control what was happening. I wanted to win. I wanted her to win. But too much damage had been done over time. We kept the chest compressions going, but the flat line on the cardiac monitor didn't budge. After several minutes I knew for sure things weren't going to change. Gloria's overworked heart just couldn't take any more. She was dead.

I never saw any of Gloria's family at the hospital, but our halls were abuzz for days about the seven-hundred-pound woman who'd been too big to leave her house. She had died in such a sad, lonely way. I wondered: Just who was she? What had happened in her life that had caused or enabled her to gain so much weight? Were there undiagnosed medical problems—perhaps an under-functioning thyroid, or an ankle or foot fracture that had contributed to her lack of mobility? Had she always been overweight? Had she experienced the breakup of a relationship or the loss of a parent that had caused a spiral into depression? Did she have friends and family who loved her unconditionally and had tried to help her?

I could only imagine how excruciating it must have been for Gloria to lie there helplessly in her own filth, unable even to wash herself properly or clip her own toenails. Long before her heart stopped, she must have felt like she was dying slowly with her eyes wide open. No one would want to live or die that way.

Gloria was the extreme, but practically every day I treat overweight black men and women—many weighing more than three hundred pounds—who are perhaps just one tragedy away from becoming her. They arrive at the E.R. with complications from diabetes, high blood pressure, or heart disease, referring to their ailments—"my sugar" or "my pressure"—as though they are old familiar belongings. For many of my patients, diabetes, high blood pressure, and heart disease indeed are very familiar. They've been handed down for generations, like family heirlooms, but at a very high cost. Nearly twice as many African Americans have diabetes, and twice as many die from heart disease and strokes, compared with our white counterparts. In most cases, the root of the problem is obesity. Eighty percent of people with diabetes are overweight. African Americans have the highest rates of obesity of all racial groups in the United States. The problem is most critical among African American women, about eighty percent of whom are overweight or obese. Scariest of all, though, are numbers showing the rate of obesity among children. Since 1980, the number of overweight children in the country has tripled. Today, about one in three children is overweight or obese. The crisis is even more severe in minority communities, where 40 percent of African American and Mexican American children are overweight or obese. In the emergency department at Beth, I regularly treated nine- and ten-year-old patients who weighed upward of 150 pounds and already showed signs of type 2 diabetes, the most common form, caused primarily by poor eating habits and lack of physical exercise. When I would consult with the mother, more times than not, she was obese, too.

There is no doubt that culture has heavily influenced this epidemic, starting perhaps with our attitudes. African Americans and Latinos tend to be more tolerant of extra weight than their white and Asian counterparts. I've always found that outlook mostly positive; it's an affirmation to black and brown girls everywhere that they can be beautiful without looking like the needle-thin, airbrushed models on magazine covers. Throughout my life, I've watched black girls grow up proudly flaunting their curves. As a black boy, I learned early that a woman with a little extra weight in all the right places is a thing of beauty. The community of brothers around me often advised, "Man, don't nobody want a bone but a dog." To this day, the most beautiful women to me have a little "meat on their bones" and some "junk in the trunk." My point: There is no one-size-fits-all standard of beauty, or perfect health, for that matter.

Still, the most universal guide to figuring out a healthy weight is the body mass index, or BMI, an adult man or woman's estimated percentage of body fat, based on the individual's height and weight. No doctor visit is necessary to get this number. Anyone with access to a computer search engine (for example, at a neighborhood library computer that provides Internet service) can plug an individual height and weight into a BMI calculator and get that important number with a few simple keyboard clicks. A BMI of 18.5 to 24.9 is considered within the normal range; from 25 to 29.9 is considered overweight; and over 30 is obese. Too often I've treated black women in the latter two categories who shrug off an unhealthy size—and thus, any attempt to do something about it—with a dismissive explanation that they are "big-boned," or "just a big girl."

Of equal concern to me, though, is research showing that weight-related attitudes and behaviors among African American and Latino women are swinging toward the opposite end of the spectrum, valuing extreme thinness over a healthy body weight. A 2001 California State University survey of 801 women and 428 men of all races found no measurable ethnic differences in how men and women viewed their own bodies and obesity in general. Women across the board were generally more dissatisfied with their bodies than men, and women of all races rated thin female shapes as more attractive than fuller shapes. Those findings were in line with separate studies in 2000 and 2003 showing that black women were as likely as white women to report binge eating and purging and even more likely than women of other races to report fasting and the abuse of laxatives and diuretics—all symptoms associated with eating disorders.

Many of our traditional soul foods—fried chicken, macaroni and cheese, pound cake, and peach cobbler, to name a few—work against a healthy lifestyle. Little black girls have stood at their mothers' and grandmothers' elbows for generations, learning how to cook with soul. That, of course, means adding ham hocks, fat-back, and lots of salt to otherwise healthy foods, such as collard greens and black-eyed peas. And our church dinners and family celebrations often center on the same spread of high-fat and highly seasoned dishes. In this age of immediate and abundant information, it should come as no surprise that many of the foods we love are loaded with artery-clogging fat. Yet there has been a major disconnect between what we know and what we do. The sad result is that we are losing our mothers, fathers, sisters, and brothers, who seem to be leading normal, busy lives when one day the unthinkable happens.

"I need a doctor now!" the nurse yelled, dashing into a patient's room where I was surrounded by a group of residents. We were nearly finished with our rounds on the observation unit for stable patients when the nurse rushed in. Working at such a busy hospital, we were accustomed to being pulled from one case to another in an emergency. We abruptly ended the discussion and scurried down the hall to another room. There we found a middle-aged woman, perhaps in her forties, sweating profusely and unresponsive. The name on her chart—Mrs. Santos—told me she was likely Latino. Her heart rate had dropped suddenly from the normal 60 to 100 beats per minute down to 20 to 25 beats, far too low for someone so young. The monitor detected an extremely high blood pressure. She was not significantly overweight, but other factors, including diet, can cause high blood pressure.

My adrenaline soared as I instructed the technician to grab the EKG machine and told the clerk to order a portable chest X-ray. My senior resident sensed the escalating crisis and jumped right in, instructing the junior resident to get the equipment for intubation. Within seconds, the junior resident had her equipment in hand and began the process. The senior resident stood over her shoulder to monitor and offer support.

In anticipation of the next step, Mike, the clerk, paged a respiratory technician, who would be needed to put the patient on a ventilator to regulate the rate and volume of oxygen flowing to her. My intern stood at Mrs. Santos's waist, inserting a large bore intravenous line through the leg to the femoral vein in the groin area. My role was to make sure the patient was receiving the best care as quickly and smoothly as possible. I moved toward the young man standing nervously in a corner of the room, presumably the patient's son, to find out what had happened. He started talking as soon as I was within earshot.

"Doc, I found her passed out in the middle of the floor this evening when I came home," he said. "When I left this morning to go to work, she was fine. She was sitting at the table having breakfast and reading her paper. I was at the counter, fixing my coffee, and she was talking about all she had to get done today.

"She asked me to drop some clothes off at the cleaners because she had to go to the bank, the supermarket, and the doctor. That was the last time I talked to her until I got home. I can't believe she was lying at home, possibly all day, without being able to move or call for help.

"Doc, what do you think is going on? She only has high blood pressure, has never smoked or drank a day in her life."

Wait. High blood pressure. "Is she on medication for the hypertension?" I asked.

"Yes," he replied. "But she doesn't like taking it. She says she doesn't like the way it makes her feel groggy and sleepy all the time. She says her pressure never makes her feel that bad, just a headache every once in a while."

Right away, I knew she'd probably had a stroke. Mrs. Santos was being rushed off to get a CAT scan, and the respiratory therapist was at the head of the bed, pumping oxygen through a bag to deliver the right amount of air to keep her vulnerable organs alive. In my mind I predicted what the scan would show: a large injured area in the brain from the stroke. But for her and her family's sake, I hoped I was wrong. I hoped she would pull through and I'd have a chance to explain to her how crucial it was that she took her medication. Her son's face showed disbelief. His eyes seemed to ask: How could this be? How could a cheerful "good morning . . . see you later for dinner" end up here? I braced myself for what I knew would be his next question: "Doc, what are her chances?"

"Well, we just have to wait and see the results of the CAT scan," I told him.

"Doc, you don't understand. I can't lose her. She is my world."

His pain was raw, and I wanted to do all I could to make things turn out right for him. But this was truly out of my hands. I excused myself and told him that I would return as soon as I had the results.

"Dr. Davis, pick up on 7240," a voice over the intercom said a few minutes later.

I reached for the phone. It was the radiologist calling with the results. The news wasn't good. Mrs. Santos had a large bleed with herniation of the brain and compression of the brain stem, explaining her low heart rate. She was basically brain dead. The life support machine was breathing for her. I returned to the room and pulled up a chair next to her son. With elbows resting on his knees, he leaned over his mother, who lay completely still in a hospital bed. The rhythmic breaths of the machine seemed louder in the silence. There is no easy way to tell someone the worst possible news about a loved one.

"I'm so sorry to tell you this," I began.

My words punctured him. I could see his hope deflating as I explained that the machines were the only thing keeping his mother alive . . . and he would have to make the painful decision of whether and when to disconnect her from them.

"Doc, you told me you would save her," he replied—wanting, at this moment surely needing, to believe that I'd actually said that.

This was grief talking. I let him vent.

"You told me she had a chance. I want you to bring her back to me, the same way she was when I left her this morning."

I took a deep breath and tried to offer some comfort. "I'm so sorry, sir. I know this isn't easy."

He dropped his head in his hands and wept.

Obesity and African Americans*

- African American women have the highest rates of being overweight or obese, compared to other groups in the United States. About four out of five African American women are overweight or obese.
- In 2009, African Americans were 1.5 times as likely to be obese as non-Hispanic whites.
- In 2009, African American women were 60 percent more likely to be obese than non-Hispanic white women.
- In 2007-2008, African American children were 30 percent more likely to be overweight than non-Hispanic whites.

HEALTH IMPACT OF OBESITY*

- More than 80 percent of people with type 2 diabetes are overweight.
- People who are overweight are more likely to suffer from high blood pressure and high levels of blood fats and LDL cholesterol—all risk factors for heart disease and stroke.
- In 2007, African Americans were 50 percent less likely to engage in active physical activity than non-Hispanic whites.
- Deaths from heart disease and stroke are almost twice the rate for African Americans as compared to whites.

For a list of free healthy weight loss tools, go to www.cdc.gov/healthyweight/tools/index .html#Family. Or contact the CDC's Division of Nutrition, Physical Activity, and Obesity at 1-800-232-4636 or TTY, 1-888-232-6348.

*Source: U.S. Department of Health and Human Services Office of Minority Health, based on statistics from the Centers for Disease Control and Prevention

13

REACHING OUT

Rhenita Oglesby was a single mother in her second year of medical school in New Jersey the day we met in 2003. She had just finished reading the memoir I'd written with Rameck and George, and she wanted to tell me her story. After a book event, I noticed her waiting patiently to speak to me, and as she introduced herself, tears filled her eyes. My success had given her hope, she said, because, like me, she had failed the first part of the state board exam that all medical students must pass to stay on the road to becoming a doctor. She had overcome so much in her life to get into medical school, but after recently failing the test, she felt her dream slipping away. I knew immediately how she felt. The memory of my own failure on the same test a few years earlier was still fresh—the panic that welled in my throat as I sat in the dean's office and received the news, the feeling of worthlessness, and the fear that all my hard work would land me short of my goal. The carrot (a medical career) was right there, dangling in front of my eyes. I could see it, smell it, and almost touch it, but I'd stumbled in my first attempt to reach for it.

My first thought: I had to help this woman. My second: Camille had been right.

I smiled to myself as I thought about Camille, a good friend and fellow medical student who had shared an apartment with Rameck and me the first year of medical school. I'd felt so alone after learning that I'd failed the state board exam that I isolated myself even more from both of my roommates, as well as from George, who was a short drive away in Newark, attending dental school. None of them could understand what I was going through, I thought. But during one of my worst moments, Camille told me: "You might not understand it now, Sam, but God allowed this to happen for a reason."

Though I appreciated Camille's attempt to comfort me, I'm certain I didn't believe her right then. She had passed the test. It was easy for her to think that God had some grand master plan for me that included what in the moment felt close to torture. But looking at the hurt in Rhenita's eyes years later, I felt instantly connected to her, and my own struggles finally seemed to make more sense. She was a stranger, but no one knew what she felt better than I. "I know what you're going through because I've been there," I told her. "And I can help you get through this."

It felt good to be able to say that to her and to stand as an example that one failure didn't have to be the end of the road for her. We exchanged contact information, and I later shared with her the advice that two of my trusted college advisers had given me to help me refocus my thoughts and energy. Before I had any chance of passing, they'd said, I had to find a way to reduce my stress. I'd been so worried about passing the test that I'd defeated myself mentally before I even sat down to take it. My advisers' words prompted me to reach back to my childhood kung fu lessons, when I'd first learned how to clear my mind through meditation. Then, slowly, I crawled out of the doldrums and began a daily routine of meditating, working out, and studying vigorously, breaking the material I needed to know for the test into digestible parts for each study session. I shut out the negative thoughts and reassured myself several times a day that I was smart enough to become a doc-tor; I just kept repeating the words to myself until I really believed them. The second time around, I passed easily. The same routine helped me pass the next two parts of the state board exam on the first try.

I shared with Rhenita the study routine that had been helpful to me, and the two of us met about once a week at the library, at Beth Israel, or at the medical school she attended. We discussed time management, outlined a plan of study, and stuck to it. We talked about the importance of her believing that she would get past this hurdle. When Rhenita took the exam a second time, she passed. Her victory felt almost as extraordinary to me as my own had. She now practices family medicine in New Jersey.

Time and time again, I found myself drawn to help other smart and hardworking young people facing some kind of chal-lenge to their dreams. I knew something about struggle. My own struggles—and finding a way to work through them—had taught me about fortitude and endurance.

After I passed my exams, and just weeks before my medical school graduation, I thought I had survived the worst and was on my way to a rewarding career, then there I was again, sitting be-fore a grim-faced dean with more bad news. None of the teaching hospitals I had applied to had chosen me for their residency pro-grams. Like every other medical student about to graduate into the real world, I had researched the teaching hospitals that offered residencies in my desired specialty (emergency medicine) and iden-tified the places where I wanted to work. I'd sent out forty applica-tions, and thirty hospitals had responded, inviting me for an interview. I'd narrowed that list to a more manageable eighteen and spent every penny I had traveling to interviews in New Jersey, New York, Washington, D.C., and Maryland, as well as in At-lanta, Cleveland, Chicago, and Philadelphia. I couldn't afford to take the train or plane to most places, so I drove to the East Coast hospitals and stayed mostly with relatives, friends, and friends of friends. I'd even schlepped through snowstorms to get to a couple of the appointments. I had just one suit, a cheap but stylish dark blue one that I'd picked up at a discount store, but I made sure it was clean for every interview. I dressed it up with a nice shirt—sky blue one time, baby blue the next. When I ranked my top choices in the National Resident Matching Program's computerized database, I was sure that at least one of my favored hospitals on the East Coast would choose me, too. But when the hospitals entered their chosen candidates into the same database, and the computer spit out the matches linking the students and hospitals, none of the hospitals on my list had chosen me. Once again, I was devastated and filled with self-doubt.

Emergency medicine is a super-competitive specialty with far more qualified applicants than slots, but I had done well academically. I couldn't help wondering: *What's wrong with me?* I will never know for sure why I didn't match, but my medical school advisers suggested that my response during a particular part of the interview certainly hadn't helped my chances; sometimes, one small detail can separate two good candidates. When questioners had asked me what I wanted to do for extracurricular activity, I'd talked about my desire to do community service. I saw more than a few puzzled looks as I sought feebly to explain the connection to medicine. I may have made a stronger impression, my advisers suggested, if I'd expressed an interest in taking classes or seminars exploring the latest in EKG or ultrasound technology, the merger of the Internet and medicine, or methods to increase patient satisfaction—all popular areas of study.

In the last-minute scramble to land a residency, I took the dean's advice and applied for a position in the more expansive field of internal medicine. I hastily accepted an offer from the University of Maryland. It was a reputable program, but I had zero interest in internal medicine. My fate seemed sealed, and I was miserable. I just kept thinking that there had to be another option, another emergency medicine residency program out there somewhere. There was no way I had come this far to be this miserable. I asked myself repeatedly: *Where do you want to be? Where would you have the best chance to shine?*

That's how I ended up a few weeks later doing another computer search of emergency medicine residency programs in New Jersey. Suddenly, Beth Israel popped up on my screen. It was the first time in all of my research that the program had surfaced. Excitement shot through me, renewing the hope that had disappeared weeks earlier. The website showed that each of the hospital's six residency slots was filled, but I didn't care. I had to know more. When I called and introduced myself, Jacquie Johnson, the hospital's residency coordinator, explained that the residency program had been revamped, expanded, and newly advertised, which was why it hadn't shown up in any of my previous searches. By the way, she added, the website had not yet been updated, and the expansion had created two additional slots in emergency medicine. I could hardly believe my ears. God had opened up the heavens and dropped this starving dog a bone. I sank my teeth in and ran with it. I immediately faxed my application and followed up with a telephone call. I got a good vibe from Jacquie. She seemed impressed that I'd grown up in Newark, and we clicked over the phone. When she told me that she would make sure to put my information into the right hands, I believed her. Sure enough, within just a few days, I was invited for an interview at the hospital.

There was something about being home again for the interview that restored my confidence. I knew this place. I knew the people. I'd sat in the same waiting room outside the E.R. at Beth Israel many times as a kid when child's play got too rough and ended in a broken bone or a gash. When the administrator showing me around the hospital opened the doors to the emergency room, I got goose bumps. This was it. Somehow, I just knew. Unlike the other interviews when I'd stumbled over my words and my insides had felt like a bowl of quivering Jell-O, I was sure that Beth Israel was the place for me. I looked my interviewers in their eyes and told them what my heart was telling me: This was where I wanted to be, where I belonged and felt confident I could thrive. After a second interview, I got an offer, and against the advice of my medical school advisers, I talked my way out of the agreement with the University of Maryland. Then, with deep gratitude, I headed home to start my career. The community service that I'd tried to make sense of in all those failed interviews made sense here. This was my community, a community filled with good kids who never make the news—kids like Kenny Malique Bazemore.

I met Malique in 2003 at a book signing event near Newark after the paperback release of *The Pact*. During the question-and-answer segment, his mother, Monica Bazemore, rose from her seat in the crowded bookstore. "I'm here because of what you've done for my son," she said, as her son, then ten, sat beside her and blushed. She explained that Malique had reminded her every day all week about the book event and had even brought pen and paper to take notes. At their home in Bloomfield, New Jersey, he had removed the sports posters on his bedroom wall and replaced them with photos of Rameck, George, and me that he had clipped from magazines. Monica asked for a few words of encouragement for Malique, but George, Rameck, and I were so touched and impressed that we got to know him and became like his big brothers. We brought him along to community events and introduced him to some of the celebrities we met, including radio host Wendy Williams and superstar Bill Cosby.

Malique was small for his age, wore glasses, and had an innocent face and an easy, shy smile. The book had inspired him to want to become a doctor, his mother said. I learned later that part of the reason he wanted to pursue a medical career was to find a cure for his then five-year-old sister, Kennedy, who had been born with a severe and rare disease of the central nervous system. Easily identified by a large mole that had grown down her face, the disease caused facial deformities and left Kennedy unable to walk, talk, or do anything for herself. After her birth, the children's father had left the family, staying in touch only sporadically, so Monica was raising both of them alone. Even at age ten, Malique had learned to help take care of his sister, handling such medical tasks as suctioning fluid from her breathing tube.

In some ways, Malique reminded me so much of myself. When I was in medical school, my desire to ease my sister Fellease's suffering from AIDS motivated me through some of my darkest days. I wanted to help him achieve his dreams. The two of us talked on the phone regularly, hung out when we could, and his mom didn't hesitate to call when he needed a little male guidance.

Once, she emailed and asked me to talk to Malique after he got into trouble at school for being disruptive in class. The next time I saw Malique, we talked about it. He told me that he was bored and that his antics—laughing and talking loudly—hadn't seemed like a big deal. I saw no need for a long speech. Malique was generally a serious kid who recognized the importance of excelling in school, keeping a clean record, and choosing his friends wisely. I just listened and told him that acting like a clown wasn't cool and that I expected more. I wanted to do for him what others had done for me: let him know that I cared, that my expectations for him were high, and that the easiest thing for him to do was behave. It was as simple as that. I knew he looked up to me and would try to meet my expectations.

By his junior year in high school, Malique was struggling. His grades had slipped, and he was no longer sure he wanted to be a doctor or even go to college. I recognized his teenage angst and rebellion and stayed close. He called me often to express his frustrations or ask for advice, and I called, emailed, and texted regularly to check in with him. I also offered moral support when he decided that he wanted to reconnect with his father. Malique located his dad in Delaware, went to live with him in his junior year, and graduated from Glasgow High School. While there, he joined the Junior Air Force ROTC, which helped him regain the discipline, organization, and focus he needed to move confidently into his future. Malique now attends Delaware State University, where he is a movement science major (similar to sports science). Though he no longer wants to be a medical doctor, he is pursuing his dream to someday have a career in medicine. He hopes to be a physical therapist to help children with special needs—like his sister—and wounded soldiers.

In my relationship with Malique and the others I mentored, I was the fortunate one. My life felt more meaningful every time I had a chance to spend time with a boy yearning for fatherly attention and affection, or to help piece together the shattered confidence of a medical student who had failed her board exams, or to offer hope to a mother raising children alone in a tough city. In them, I saw the huge difference that one person can make in another's life. I could offer healing and perhaps even help save lives (and dreams) beyond the emergency room. Maybe inspiring a kid to go to college or to get serious about school could even lessen the chances that I'd see him down the road in the emergency room with a bullet in him. Inspiring kids to dream bigger than what they could see was exactly our hope when George, Rameck, and I established The Three Doctors Foundation in April 2000. When the three of us returned home to Newark-area hospitals for our residencies, newspaper stories about the friendship that had helped three poor inner-city boys become doctors resulted in speaking invitations throughout the region. We were giddy for the opportunity to share our story, and rather unexpectedly we amassed about $3,000 in gifts from those engagements. That was a lot of cash to us. I had returned to Newark with less than $30 to my name and, despite being a doctor, was still trying to get past living from paycheck to paycheck. But each of us felt a tremendous need to use the money to create something that would benefit the community. Many people had given of their time and resources to us along our journey, and we wanted to give some of it back, even though we didn't know if we'd ever have that kind of extra cash again.

At first, we talked about giving the money away as a college scholarship to a needy, deserving student, but then what? The more we talked, the more we realized we wanted to do something more expansive, more hands-on. We wanted to give kids in neighborhoods like the ones where we grew up what we didn't have: close and personal access to the array of professionals out there—doctors, nurses, lawyers, accountants, business owners, and others who could share their paths and offer one-on-one guidance. We could sponsor fun events to bring them all together, raise money for scholarships, and use our expertise in the medical field to educate the community about the array of medical problems killing us disproportionately. Kids might walk away from our events still believing they were the next Jay-Z or Kobe (and who knows, maybe they are), but we could show them early on that they had options.

George, Rameck, and I were by far the poorest philanthropists we knew, but at least we had a structure and a little cash in place for a small grassroots operation. We began mentioning the foundation in speeches, and volunteers stepped forward to help us get set up legally, establish a website, and plan events. One of our first big activities was Mentor Day, where we recruited professionals from all over the community and matched them as closely as possible with students who had similar aspirations—the boy who dreamed of opening a business someday and the CEO; the girl who played school with her baby dolls and the real live teacher; the kid who was good with numbers and the accountant; the poor student who never thought college was a possibility and the university counselor.

For another of the foundation's events, the Positive Peer Pressure Challenge, Malique placed among the winners. The purpose of the challenge was to flip the way peer pressure usually works by rewarding young people who were positively influencing their peers. We asked students to write in and tell us about their efforts, and we awarded prizes—laptops to the top winners and iPods and gaming systems to those who placed second and third place. Malique had volunteered at a nursing home and chronicled his experience poignantly with photos and a journal. For his efforts, he won his first laptop.

I'll never forget another of the foundation's events, its first Healthy Mind and Body Summit on July 3, 2003. It was held at the Boys and Girls Club on the same block where my parents first lived when they moved to Newark. The event drew about five hundred people throughout the day for a roster of activities that included free blood pressure and diabetes screenings, guest speakers on a variety of motivational and health topics, as well as live performances. Among the most memorable were three little dudes, ages from thirteen to fifteen, who dressed up like George, Rameck, and me, in white lab coats over their sagging jeans and T-shirts, and did an original rap to one of rapper 50 Cent's beats. But they weren't boasting about criminal exploits, degrading women, or dogging one another. They were telling another kind of story:

> *I don't know what you heard about the*
> *Three doctors from the Brick City*
> *George Jenkins, Rameck Hunt, and Sam D . . .*

It was so much fun to watch them, full of energy and enthusi-asm, delivering their own interpretation of our message that edu-cation is the most permanent way off the streets. Their performance earned them their own fan club. Swooning girls wanted to take pictures with them. And I walked away feeling great, thinking, *These little dudes get it. They really heard us.*

Young people like the teen rappers I met that day are why I—and all of us who want to be part of finding solutions to the vio-lence and health crises in our country—can't give up. We know that young people are listening and watching. And we believe that when we provide them with the information they need to make responsible choices and help them to recognize their own power, we save lives.

14

UNEXPECTED TWISTS

Though I grew up less than a half hour away from it, New York City seemed about as distant as the Milky Way. It didn't matter that Newark sat just on the other side of the Hudson River. After struggling every day to make ends meet, my parents didn't have the money, the time, or the inclination to take us kids sightseeing in the Big Apple. As a boy, I never stood at the Statue of Liberty, saw the lights on Broadway, or strolled through Central Park. The first time I ventured to Times Square, I was in high school. My older sister Fellease, my brother Andre, and their spouses at the time allowed me to tag along one cold winter evening when they took the train into the city. I tried to play it cool, to pretend that the skyscrapers, bright lights, and fast-moving crowds didn't faze me. But on the inside I was like a giddy elementary-school kid, savoring every minute of his first field trip. Everything seemed larger, brighter, and faster than I'd imagined.

By the time I finally made it to Radio City Music Hall, I was twenty-seven and nearly a year into my residency at Beth Israel. *Essence* magazine had chosen George, Rameck, and me to receive its 2000 Lifetime Achievement Award. I was crazy excited about the award, not just because of who was singling us out—*Essence* magazine, one of the premier black publications—but also because of what this recognition represented. Three young doctors would be center stage before a star-studded crowd on national television alongside the community's much-heralded music, entertainment, and sports idols. This would definitely help with our foundation's goal of glamorizing education and bringing academic stars out of hiding, particularly in urban schools where wannabe pro athletes and rappers reign. The ceremony didn't disappoint. Suddenly, my family and I were right in the middle of the New York glitz that I'd only seen on TV. It had been tough trying to decide how to divvy up the tickets among my family and closest friends, but in the end I was joined by my mother and father; my father's wife, Thelma; my brother Andre and his wife, Makeba; my lifelong friend Will (whose daughter is my godchild); and my then-girlfriend. I sent limos to pick up my family, and I don't think I'd ever seen my father, all five feet nine inches of him, walk as tall as he did into Radio City Music Hall that night. He was beaming, and my mother couldn't stop saying how proud she was of me. There we were, the Davis clan, breathing the same air as Bill Cosby and Oprah Winfrey.

I'd wanted Fellease to be there, but by then she was too sick. She had, however, felt well enough to help Moms prepare for the event. The two of them had gone shopping together, and for a rare moment, they were just mother and daughter, enjoying life in its simplicity, without the angst caused by addiction and disease. The two of them chose a pants suit—a white evening jacket with black slacks—for Moms, who relished the fact that Fellease had arranged a hair appointment for her. "You know your sister picked out my outfit, helped me with my makeup, and made me get my hair done," she bragged to me that night—this from a woman who would choose to wear a wig over her own hair any day.

When Fellease died the next year, I dropped by to see Moms one summer day and was stunned to find her bald. She had shaved off every inch of her hair. She read the shock in my eyes and responded before I could even speak: "It was too hot, Marshall, and so I had to cut it off," she said matter-of-factly. To this day, I believe that this small act was her way of regaining control of her life after Fellease's death. I'm no psychologist, but I know this: Moms couldn't do a thing about her daughter's addiction, or the suffering it caused, or the AIDS that finally killed her, but it was hot, and her hair was sweaty, and she didn't want to be bothered with hot, sweaty hair, and she certainly *could* do something about that.

The *Essence* award opened my world a bit wider. Oprah's producers called, and Rameck, George, and I later appeared on her show, as well as the *Today* show. Radio hosts Tavis Smiley and Tom Joyner also interviewed us on their top-rated black radio programs. Our memoir became a bestseller, and we began sharing our story all over the country, from classrooms to corporate boardrooms to auditoriums. Our foundation grew, attracting the volunteers needed to carry out our mentoring and scholarship programs. My social life got an upgrade, too. I no longer had to talk my way behind the ropes to many of the A-list parties and hot spots, which was, quite frankly, intoxicating to a young single doctor who'd made it his mission to explore the New York he'd missed as a child. New York became my escape from the stress of work. After a long, mentally exhausting shift, I'd dash home, shower and change, grab some food on the run, and make my way through the Holland Tunnel into Manhattan. Often, I'd party until the wee hours of morning, racing the sunrise to get home. I'd sleep three or four hours and then head back to the hospital to start all over again. I didn't need much sleep—at least, that's what I told myself.

So there I was one winter night, at the Soho Grand Hotel for pop star Mariah Carey's surprise birthday party. I looked up, and Denzel was on my left and music mogul L. A. Reid on my right. Still new to these types of events, I played it cool, mingling like I belonged in this glamorous crowd. But every now and then, when I saw another familiar famous face, I had the urge to rush over and say, "Hey, I'm a big fan of your work! May I have your autograph?"

As usual, I hung out until just before sunrise, and then started the half-hour drive home. I did everything I could to overpower the desire to sleep—danced in the car, bopping up and down on my seat, and sang out loud. I even rolled down the windows and stuck my face into the frigid air. I made it home safely, but in three hours, I was up again, racing to the hospital for the Wednesday morning lecture, where residents learn the meat and grit of the E.R. I returned home for lunch, changed into my scrubs, and went back to work for an overnight shift. Staying alert during those twelve hours—well, let's just say it was a challenge. At about 2.00 A.M., I entered a room to check on a patient who had complained of a migraine. The room was dark to help ease the patient's pain, and she was asleep. I nudged her, and she moaned, "Leave me alone." I tried again, and she uttered her demand even more forcefully.

I pulled a plastic chair to her bedside with the intent to take her medical history, and then spoke loudly to get her attention. She muttered a few more choice words, and that's all I remember. The next thing I knew, I heard voices. I opened my eyes to find practically the entire emergency department staff, including my boss, surrounding me, staring, with worry in their eyes. Somehow, the dark room, the patient's refusal to wake up, and my exhaustion had caused me to crash right there. It was too late to pretend to carry on with business as usual. I was busted. Then, for some strange reason, the whole scene just seemed funny. I mumbled something about keeping my patient company and burst out laughing hysterically. My colleagues joined in. I guess they were relieved to know I was only sleeping.

Fortunately, the residency director took it all in stride and didn't say a word. I'd never stumbled before that point, and my work ethic was not in question. But I didn't need a reprimand to know that my body and mind had reached their limits. As a doctor, I should have known better. The medical community has long debated the effects of sleep deprivation among medical residents, who traditionally work excessive hours (without even considering personal factors that can exacerbate the issue). Numerous reports have shown that lack of sleep harms physicians' job performance and increases the potential for medical errors. A few years later, in 2003, the Accreditation Council for Graduate Medical Education would revise its guidelines, including an eighty-hour cap on the maximum weekly hours young doctors can work, but permitting shifts up to thirty hours. Critics argued that the changes did not go far enough. A congressional probe would ultimately push the council, in 2011, to implement more changes, including a maximum sixteen-hour work shift, followed by at least eight hours off, for residents. And the debate over further guidelines continues.

Before these new rules and my own literal wake-up call, I was like many busy people who think they don't need much sleep to function well. I now know better. While it is true that the amount of sleep a person needs is as individual as the person, the National Sleep Foundation estimates that the average healthy man or woman needs between seven and nine hours a night. Too little sleep (generally six hours or less) slows reaction time and impairs vision and judgment, which can result in tragic consequences, particularly on the road. Drowsy drivers cause more than 100,000 motor vehicle accidents each year, 1,550 of them resulting in death and another 71,000 in injuries, according to the National Highway Traffic Safety Administration. Studies also show that staying awake for more than twenty hours can cause impairment equal to that of a person considered legally drunk.

I was lucky. I never caused any accidents on the road, my patient didn't wake up during my ordeal, and the rest of that fateful night was relatively slow. But I resolved then that it would never happen again. I couldn't continue at the same pace. I had to achieve greater balance in my life, and making sure I got enough sleep was a huge part of that.

The other part was figuring out how to balance the demands of my work life with what had become my equal passion: community service. I was certain that reaching beyond the hospital walls to share with young people a message of self-empowerment could in the long run save as many lives as my work inside the emergency room. Problem was, time. I never had enough of it. Whenever the weekly schedule was sent out, I began calling my colleagues to try to negotiate a shift swap so that I could make it to a foundation event or speaking engagement. My co-workers were accommodating when they could be, but I worried how long their patience would last. That's what pushed me into Darrell Terry's office with a proposal one day in 2002.

In any profession, it's always good to know somebody among the higher-ups who has your back. For me, that was Darrell Terry, then vice president of operations at Beth Israel. He was in his late thirties when we met in 2000, and I quickly connected to him as a friend and mentor. From my early days of residency, he looked after me and made sure I knew that his door was always open to me. I took those words literally and many times walked in unannounced just to chat. His office was on the hospital's main floor, in the administrative suite, which housed all of the executives' offices. An assistant sat just inside the suite to greet guests and announce a visitor to the appropriate administrator. I often walked in, greeted her, and kept on trekking toward Darrell's office. Sometimes, the assistant would stop me mid-stride: "Mr. Terry is in a meeting. Would you like him to call the E.R.?" A short time later,

Darrell would make his way to my department, and if things were quiet, we'd catch up on the goings-on at the hospital, sports, and our personal lives. I admired that at the time he was a single father raising his son and daughter (though he would tell me later that he was uncomfortable with the well-intentioned praise he got from so many people for doing what he considered his responsibility).

Darrell had grown up nearby in East Orange, and, like me, had been born at Beth Israel. We both felt strongly that the hospital should be more than just a place where people worked, that it had an obligation to give back to the poor community that sustained it. But with a bachelor's degree in business and a master's in healthcare administration, Darrell was also a company man. He had taken the traditional route up the corporate ladder, where the gray-haired guy passes you the torch after you've spent time in the trenches earning your stripes, and he was determined to help me understand the way things worked. When I talked with him about my desire to move up quickly at the hospital, he urged patience. Slow down, I had my entire career ahead of me, he advised. That's mostly how we differed. I felt an urgency to get things done right away, to move up so that I would be in a position to help direct some of the hospital's resources into improving the surrounding community. As I saw it, the community needed us now. The Legends, Snakes, and Debras out there kept showing up in the E.R., day after day, shot up, beaten up, and damaged beyond repair. What if it was part of my job to find ways to help the hospital reach beyond the confines of its own walls and into the surrounding community?

That's the idea I posed to Darrell during a conversation one day. He was intrigued. From a strictly business point of view it made sense for the hospital to use me in that way. The 2002 publication of *The Pact* had raised my profile dramatically. There were constant requests for interviews, and cameras began following me around the hospital so often that some of my co-workers jokingly called me "Dr. Hollywood." Beth Israel was a natural part of my narrative, which brought it into the public eye. Darrell joked that hospitals more often got that kind of publicity when they cut off the wrong leg. He promised to talk to his bosses to see what they could work out.

Shortly after my residency ended on July 1, 2002, Darrell called me into his office to share the good news: I had been promoted to part-time director of community outreach. While I would continue in my role as an attending physician in the emergency department, seven hours of my workweek could be devoted to community work. There was no detailed job description, which was great because it allowed me the flexibility to define the position. I was ecstatic. The protected hours eased my schedule somewhat, allowing me to do some of my community speaking engagements on company time. But I also helped to create new programs, like an anti-smoking campaign that included therapy and a support group for men and women who were addicted to nicotine. They met regularly at the hospital and shared their challenges and triumphs. I also became the go-to guy when high schools and colleges brought student groups to the hospital. I talked to students, often over lunch, about how Beth Israel had changed the course of my life and how they, too, could achieve their dreams. Interested students shadowed me in the emergency room, and I took part in the hospital's annual Black History Month celebration honoring a local hero.

I also participated in the hospital's yearly event that brought together the families of organ donors with the patients who received their loved one's organs. There was always such joy in the room among those who got a second chance at life and the family members who got to see at least a part of their loved ones live on. The program inspired me to remember every time I renewed my driver's license to check the box agreeing to become an organ donor (and to let my family members know my wishes) if I happened to meet an untimely end. It was a commitment that I'd first made in medical school, and it's a simple way that each of us can have a profound impact on another person's life.

I'm a strong believer in partnerships, and Beth Israel seemed to me a natural partner for The Three Doctors Foundation, especially for two of our signature community events, Mentor Day and the Healthy Mind and Body Summit. For Mentor Day, hospital volunteers are matched with Newark children interested in medical careers. For the summit, hospital staff and medical students are provided with free blood pressure screenings, literature, and lectures about heart disease, diabetes, sexually transmitted infections, obesity, prostate and breast cancer, smoking cessation, depression, and other issues that have a significant (and often disproportionate) impact on minority communities. One of my favorite events as community outreach director was the hospital's annual holiday celebration that provided gifts donated by hospital employees to poor families in the community. I loved this event so much because I'd never forgotten how much a similar celebration had once meant to my family and me.

I was about eight years old that blustery winter day when my mother, Andre, Carlton, and I hopped on the number 24 public bus and headed downtown to the Newark Symphony Hall for a Christmas party thrown by strangers. My mother signed us in, and we took our seats among the crowd of families already gathered there. Holiday music played in the background, and then I heard someone announce, "The Davis family." My mother grabbed Carlton's hand and mine, and we all walked to the stage. The presenter handed Moms a big black plastic bag filled with brand-new toys and clothes. Andre, Carlton, and I were so excited that we wanted to rip into the bag right there. But my mother thanked the presenter, and we rode the bus back home and put the gifts under our Christmas tree. I felt like I was about to pop with anticipation every time I walked past that pile of gifts—that year, I felt like a normal kid. I'd been embarrassed during the holiday season in previous years when other kids talked about the new bikes, Big Wheels, and board games they were getting for Christmas, and I had nothing to share. Now some stranger had given us a Christmas. I never forgot that feeling.

Hospital administrators threw their full support behind me in my new role. They lent staff and financial support and showed up at community events to mingle with our neighbors. I was still as busy as ever, spending far more than seven hours a week volunteering in the community, but transferring seven of those hours into my workweek lessened the load a bit and increased my sense of fulfillment. The experience taught me a valuable life lesson: Ask for what you want on the job, and increase the chances of a positive response by presenting the mutual benefits.

I was in a good place mentally when a friend invited me to a house party in Brooklyn in July 2003. Brooklyn had not impressed me the few times I'd visited before, but something about the atmosphere seemed different that day as I made my way through the Holland Tunnel, across the Manhattan Bridge, and down Flatbush and DeKalb Avenues, finally landing at a two-story brick house in a tree-shrouded neighborhood.

The girls seemed earthier; the guys more laid back. I liked this vibe. Music blasted through the house, and a nice breeze kept the humidity and mosquitoes at bay. A DJ set up in the corner of the backyard played a crazy mix of the hottest songs. I was really digging the scene when I looked up and noticed a beautiful young lady standing a few feet away. She stood about five feet five inches tall, with curly, shoulder-length brown hair, a golden honey complexion, a knockout smile, and the body to match. Dressed in a fitted red T-shirt, low-cut dark blue jeans, and stilettos, she was waiting in line for the bathroom. As I watched her move forward in line, I came up with a plan to meet her: I would ease closer, wait for her to step out of the restroom, and make my move. On cue, just a few minutes later, she sauntered out, heading directly toward me. Suddenly she was close enough to touch. Palms sweating, heart pounding, I tried to think of something smooth to say, but my mind went blank. That's the only excuse I have to explain the cheesy line that came flying out: "Hey, could I have some of that?"

I was referring to an oversized plastic cup she was holding in her hand, and I immediately wanted to freeze the moment, rewind, and start over. She looked at me as if to say, *Honey, please! Try again.* And she walked away.

About a half hour later, I got another chance when I noticed her standing next to celebrity publicist Marvet Britto, whom I'd recently met. I asked her about her friend.

"Oh, you mean Melissa," Marvet responded.

My red T-shirt, stiletto-wearing friend now had a name. When Marvet introduced us, Melissa, who worked with the American Black Film Festival, first gave me that "Oh, the guy with the whack line" stare. But she quickly warmed. We talked for about a half hour, exchanged numbers, and I called her the next day. Thus began my falling in love—with Melissa, who later became a creative director at a national magazine, and with Brooklyn.

Her neighborhood was a jazzy, diverse place with people of all races and immigrants from around the world. Trees lined the streets, and there wasn't a mall or chain store in sight. The commercial establishments were primarily small specialty shops, corner diners, and other eateries, with names like Sugarcane, Mike's, and Buttercup. People actually sat outside, and they even talked and looked out for one another. There were basketball courts filled with little Kobes shooting hoops. When you walked the streets, strangers smiled and greeted you. This wasn't some cookie-cutter suburb, like the one in South Jersey where I'd lived during medical school.

Back then, my apartment was in a huge complex, where little more than Sheetrock separated me from people I never saw. By day, they vanished (probably to Philly to work); I found it so strange to see rows and rows of parked cars every day and no human beings, ever. In the evenings and on weekends, I'd hear televisions, music, and voices, the only evidence I had that people actually lived within those walls. And God forbid you ever got stuck in the elevator with a real live person. There seemed to be some kind of unwritten rule against saying hello. People would rather stare at the back of your head than actually face you to say good morning. Needless to say, that was not my vibe. Brooklyn, however, had a pulse.

Before I knew it, months turned into years. And I was still digging Brooklyn and Melissa. Life was settling into a good place.

The rumors started swirling around the E.R. in 2004: Big budget cuts were coming to Beth, and my part-time position as director of community outreach was on the chopping block. I went to Darrell Terry to get the truth. Always straight up with me, Darrell confirmed what I feared, that the tight budget would likely squeeze out my position. The hospital appreciated my work and connections to the community, he said, but tough financial times demanded difficult choices. He would do what he could to protect the hours, but he couldn't make any promises.

I then turned to Dr. Marc Borenstein, chairman of the emergency medicine department. He, too, said he'd try to prevent the hours from being cut. Dr. B, as we called him, was one of the coolest white dudes I'd ever met. He played the guitar and didn't mind showing off his dance moves at staff parties. We had shared some meaningful conversations, during which he talked about his own struggles growing up. Struggle can leave a lifelong imprint on a person's soul, and it often breeds compassion. Dr. B was a compassionate soul and one of my biggest supporters. This budget issue, though, was out of his hands.

For months I met with every administrator I knew, including executive director Paul Mertz, to try to save the position, but the inevitable happened—it was cut. To avoid a loss in pay, I would have to return to working full-time in the emergency department. The news was deeply disappointing. I could hardly fathom how seven measly hours a week of community time would even register in the size of the budget needed to operate a major urban medical center with more than six hundred beds. There had to be more to it than I was hearing. I wondered: Was it me? What had I done but try to connect the place to the community, save some lives, and bring the spotlight to a gritty urban hospital that had helped a native son rise? What about the things all the higher-ups had told me about the hospital's commitment to the community? For once I felt out of sync with Beth Israel. And that hurt.

I knew I couldn't return to the chaos of my life in the emergency department before the change, so I began negotiating with the administrators to come up with an alternative that would be cost-effective for the hospital and still allow me the time I needed physically and mentally to continue trying to make a difference in my community. We considered the possibility of trying to secure grant funding for the position, but that quickly fell through, given that I had no time to write a proposal or assistant to help me. We also talked briefly about possibly merging The Three Doctors Foundation with Beth Israel, but George, Rameck, and I decided that it was important to remain independent. I wanted things to work out at Beth, but it seemed that our talks kept leading nowhere.

In the middle of negotiations, I traveled to the nation's capital to attend the annual American College of Emergency Physicians conference, where I reconnected with a colleague I'd first met years earlier. I had just begun my residency at Beth Israel when several people told me that I needed to meet Dr. Duane J. Dyson. He'd grown up in East Orange, a small city on the border of Newark, and returned home to work at East Orange General Hospital, where he quickly made his way up to chairman of the emergency department. I called and arranged to meet him at his hospital. The first time I saw him, I was immediately struck by his presence. He was a cool, confident African American man in his late thirties. As he showed me around his department, I was impressed by how he seemed so in control. He had a comfortable, down-to-earth manner with both patients and staff. This was the kind of doctor I wanted to be.

The two of us talked for about an hour, and I identified with him as he talked passionately about how he had returned home to make a difference in his community. With a population of nearly 70,000 residents at the time, East Orange struggled with the same social problems—drugs, gangs, and violent crimes—as its bigger next-door neighbor. Dr. Dyson had heard my story and thought I would be an asset to his team. When I was done with my training, he'd said, I could have a job with him. That was an exciting prospect, and I kept it in the back of my mind, even though at the time I couldn't envision leaving Beth.

When I ran into Dr. Dyson again at the medical conference, he told me that he'd been busy creating a new organization. Drug and gang violence had continued to grow and spread in East Orange, and he was tired of seeing so many young men and women, mostly black and Latino youths, come through his emergency room with gunshots and stab wounds. With financing from the New Jersey attorney general's office and private donors, he'd created

the Violence Prevention Institute, a non-profit organization pro-
viding gang and drug prevention programs to young people and
educating the adults in their lives. I was particularly intrigued by
an initiative called "Cops and Docs," a kind of *Scared Straight!*
model that would present kids with an unglamorized look at the
consequences of gang and drug violence: no Hollywood lights
and soundtracks, just police officers discussing the sights, sounds,
and smells of death and dying; pictures depicting the mangled and
bloody faces and body parts encountered at the scene after a gun
battle; emergency room doctors sharing an unflinching look at
what it takes to patch someone back together after a knifing or
shooting, even including the scary-looking surgical tools; and a
real gunshot victim talking about what it was like to lie in your
own blood on the street, unable to move or control your bodily
functions. The description of the program blew me away. I promised to call him to learn more after the conference ended and we
were both back in New Jersey.

Meanwhile, I was still hopeful that Beth and I would be able to
reach an agreement. Months of back-and-forth talks had yielded
nothing definitive. Then one day in December 2004, I joined Rameck and George at a local gym for our foundation's annual
"Spirit of Giving" holiday event—a charity basketball game and a
clothing, food, and toy drive that enabled us to bring the joy of
Christmas to dozens of poor families. Corporate donors brought
checks for thousands of dollars to support the effort, and community members brought enough wrapped gifts and non-perishable
food to fill the room's many tables. All sat down together for a
holiday feast, the gift giveaway, and the basketball game, featuring
the three of us and guest players against a team of volunteers. At
the end of a long but gratifying Saturday, I was ready to rest, but
that was not possible. I had to report to Beth for the night shift.

Weeks earlier, when the schedule for December had been sent

out, I'd noticed that I'd been assigned to work on the same day as The Three Doctors Foundation event, and I emailed the scheduler to request the day off. There was nothing she could do, she said, but she encouraged me to try to find another doctor to cover for me. I knew the chance of finding a colleague willing to work an overnight shift on a Saturday for me was about as likely as winning the lottery. I was stuck.

That night, as I stepped out of my car just moments before I was due to report for my nine-hour shift, and a mere hour after the charity event had ended, the frigid air seemed colder than I remembered. I buttoned my leather coat all the way to the top and slid the strap of my briefcase onto my shoulder. The air turned to smoke every time I exhaled. Winter was off to a brutal start. As I walked slowly across the parking lot, everything felt heavier than usual—my bag, the air, every step I took. I whispered to myself: *"I can't do this anymore."* Between work, the foundation, travel, and all that came with sharing my message with the world, I was just plain tired. The way I saw it, my opportunity to reach the hip-hop and younger generations eye-to-eye would last only so long. Even though I was by then approaching thirty-two, I looked younger than my years. I could see in their eyes that they didn't view me as some elder with no understanding of what they were going through, preaching down to them from a bully pulpit. They knew my story. My struggle was theirs. If I made it, they could, too. I was them.

Something had to give. I called Dr. Dyson.

By mid-2005, Melissa and I were spending every spare moment together, hanging out at events in New York City or Brooklyn or relaxing at her place. I'd begun to feel that it was finally time for me to move out of the Jacksons' home and find a place of my own. I'd never considered living anywhere but Newark, but when I heard about an available condo in South Orange, my old Seton Hall stomping ground, I decided to take a look. It was spacious, modern, and just a short train ride into the city. The surrounding community was more diverse than I remembered, the neighborhood was familiar, and I liked the feel of a college town. Reluctant to buy the first place I saw, I looked at other places, both inside Newark and in surrounding areas. Nothing else measured up. I felt guilty at first about even thinking of living outside of my city, but that feeling soon passed. Newark had been my world, and I reassured myself that there was nothing wrong with branching out. I wasn't abandoning my hometown; it was ingrained in my heart and soul. And I would never stop working to make it better.

I bought the property in May, and it felt good to claim my small piece of the American dream. I took my time outfitting the place with furniture and moved in the following July. A short time later, Melissa and I agreed that she should move in with me. We both knew our relationship was for keeps.

By then, I'd also begun a new professional adventure. A job offer had come a few months earlier from Dr. Dyson, inviting me to join his new Violence Prevention Institute. The plan was for me to reach kids primarily through the Institute's "Cops and Docs" program and spend the other half of my time working under contract in the emergency rooms at two hospitals, St. Michael's Medical Center in Newark and Raritan Bay in Perth Amboy. The emergency department at Raritan Bay was run by Dr. Joe Calabro and Dr. Dane Clarke, vice chairman of the Institute, and the balance between clinical duties and community work seemed perfectly aligned with my goals and vision. Dr. Dyson was doing something different, and I was excited to be part of it. Saying yes had been easy. Letting go of Beth was the difficult part.

I'd always figured I'd be one of those Beth Israel employees who hung around long enough to get my gold pen and watch. On the distant day of my retirement, my decades of service would be emblazoned on a plaque. Speakers would regale the audience with tales of how I took my first breath within these walls, got my first stitches and cast there, and how I passed the imposing tan brick structure every day on the 107 and 39 public buses as I made my way to and from University High School. My brother Andre would surely want to talk about the time when I was about six years old, and he received a butt-whipping on my behalf when I got hurt after he finally allowed me to tag along with him to a park. I'd taken it on myself to try to fix a broken old bench, and a concrete slab twice my weight toppled over, crushing my foot. My parents blamed Andre for not watching me closely enough and rushed me off to Beth.

Maybe someone would tell the story of the afternoon when I strolled onto the bike path at Weequahic Park and collided with a bike rider, whose handlebars knocked out my front baby teeth. And back to Beth we went. And, of course, there was the night in high school when I stumbled around outside the emergency room ambulance bay with my friends after one of them smoked marijuana for the first time and thought he was dying. The audience would get a good laugh, knowing all had ended well. The accident-prone, mischievous boy who'd grown into a troubled teenager had returned home to Beth as a doctor, and spent his life there trying to save others. The end.

That's the storybook finale that had played out many times in my head.

It wasn't supposed to change abruptly on an ice-cold morning in January 2005, just six years into my career at Beth, with me sitting in Dr. B's office, silently rehearsing how I'd break the news that it was time for me to leave. When I'd first begun considering my life without Beth, I'd reached out to the University of Medicine and Dentistry of New Jersey in Newark and even got close to an agreement to work as an E.R. doctor there. Like Beth, it was familiar, and that was comforting. I'd spent countless hours doing trauma rotations there during residency. Its reputation for saving lives after a trauma was unmatched in our area. If you had eight minutes to live and were five minutes from another hospital and ten minutes from University, you would want to take the gamble to try to get to University. The place was just that good. It's funny, though, that during my childhood we always joked that "UMDNJ" stood for U Most Die in New Jersey. Perhaps that was because many of the gunshot victims from the neighborhood were taken there, and many never made it out. I suppose it was just easier to joke about the perceived inadequacies of the hospital rather than face the difficult truth about why so many black boys never made it home. But I saw close-up that University had the staff, the know-how, and the equipment to mobilize like nowhere else when a life was on the line. The thing that concerned me, though, was that there was no structured community outreach program at University, and while the hospital's administrators said all the right things to woo me, I feared I would end up in the same situation I'd found at Beth.

So there I was before Dr. B, and it was showtime. When I finally said aloud the words I'd rehearsed to myself, they didn't come as a huge shock to him. From our earlier talks, he'd gauged that I was unhappy. He and I both knew it was time for me to move on. As I stood to leave, Dr. B walked from behind his oversized desk and gave me a hug. He said he understood my decision and knew it had been a tough one for me. He wished me well. A few days later, I sent in the official letter of resignation, but I kept my leaving quiet, telling only my closest associates and swearing them to secrecy. Walking away would be tough enough. I didn't want any prolonged good-byes.

The three months seemed to rush past, and as the time wound

down, I found myself thinking about the lives I'd saved, the many I'd lost, the laughs, the learning, the frustrations, the joy, the tears I'd shared with so many within these walls. The day before my last shift, I was sitting at the desk typing a note about a patient when an EMS worker rolled in with a man who had been found wandering the Newark airport. The patient carried no bags, had no personal belongings, and appeared to be in a confused stupor. The only items that emergency workers had found in his pockets were a ticket to Mexico and some local telephone numbers. One of the residents that I was supervising picked up the man's chart while I talked to the emergency crew.

"Dr. Davis, I can't believe you're leaving," Rob, one of the emergency technicians, said. "We need you to stay."

The word was out.

I thought about my mother, who had told me many times throughout my life that I should always grow, reach new heights, and never hold myself back. I often drew inspiration from her. She rarely addressed an issue directly—as in, "Yes, son, it's a good idea for you to leave," or "No, son, I think you should stay." She'd just throw out one of her sayings and leave it to me to extract the meaning. I was stepping into the unknown, but I knew I shouldn't be afraid to grow.

The resident approached our airport patient and completed a medical history and a physical. She was now ready to explain her findings to me. In her confident second-year voice, the young doctor presented her case. The patient was confused and appeared to have an altered mental status. His vital signs were normal, but he had some abrasions on his head and scalp swelling. Otherwise, his exam was benign. I listened, and then asked for her diagnosis before chiming in. She named five possible medical conditions. Then she added that she wanted to call the telephone numbers found in the patient's pocket. I smiled. This was a simple but key step that set apart the great clinicians. One extra step could go a long way in figuring out a case. She had learned well, and I would miss this part of my job.

I had told no one in the department when my final day would be, and so I was surprised to see my co-workers appear with a cake in my final moments. We then gathered in the break room to say our good-byes. They had taught me so much, and I was grateful. There is no harder-working, more talented group of people any-where. But I felt none of the sadness and emotion that I'd experi-enced when the decision was new. I felt only peace. I packed my things, slid on my leather jacket, pulled my bag onto my shoulder, and waved one last farewell. As I stepped into the parking lot, there were no fireworks, just the nippy air and a knowing in my soul:

Beth would be fine. And so would I.

AFTERWORD

My work at the Violence Prevention Institute put me right where I wanted to be: in kids' faces with the truth. And there was no better partner than my colleague Hashim Garrett, a former gang member who was fifteen years old in May 1990, when he learned firsthand what it was like to get shot. Hashim, partially paralyzed from the waist down, would make his way to the front of a room slowly, using metal crutches strapped across his wrists. Then he'd share his spellbinding story: How six bullets from a Tec-9 semi-automatic handgun tore through his flesh, striking his spinal cord, leaving him unable to move or control his bodily functions. How he lay under an elevated train track on the streets of Brooklyn for the longest half hour of his life, waiting for help and pleading with God not to let him die. How he spent six grueling months in the hospital, unable at first even to go to the bathroom without help.

Then I'd feed off Hashim, pull from my medical bag the tools of emergency medicine, including a scary-looking scalpel and a gigantic "rib spreader," which is used to crack open the chest during surgery. I'd describe how a Foley catheter is inserted to drain urine from the body and how a plastic "poop bag" collects feces outside the body when the intestines no longer work. I'd show pictures of real gunshot victims, surgical procedures and damaged organs, then reveal how the once-tough drug dealers and gang members, riddled with bullet holes, cried for their mamas and pleaded with me to save their lives once they got to the emergency room.

The Institute's team included other board-certified emergency medicine physicians, a social worker, and Hashim. Our presentations were explicitly graphic; we got the kids' attention. I could see it in their eyes and hear it in their torrent of questions. We frightened some of them, too, but in this situation, fear was a good thing. We wanted kids to fear drugs, gangs, and guns enough to stay away from them. We showed our young audiences the real life-altering and deadly consequences of bad choices, but we also provided information and training to help them make smarter ones. From 2005 to 2007, I visited at least eighty elementary, middle, and high schools in Newark, East Orange, West Orange, and Irvington. The work was therapeutic, powerful, and purposeful. Unfortunately, though, it did not last. The program had been funded primarily by a two-year grant from the office of then New Jersey Attorney General Peter C. Harvey, but the funds were not renewed after Harvey left office in 2006. The news was extremely disappointing, especially given that our politicians spend many millions on the back end of violence, treating gunshot victims in hospitals and housing the perpetrators in jails.

It is impossible to provide raw data showing how many students rejected gangs or drug deals or walked away from potentially deadly arguments because of what they'd learned and experienced through the Institute, but I have no doubt that we changed minds and hearts and saved lives. In financial terms, even if we prevented just one child from getting shot, we saved the state of New Jersey tens of thousands of dollars. The medical costs of treating just one serious gunshot patient, including hospitalization, were then an estimated $300,000. Meanwhile, the Institute operated on a

$400,000 grant for two years. After its primary source of financing was eliminated, though, the Institute cut staff and scaled back dramatically.

I left the program in 2007 with tremendous admiration for my former colleagues, particularly Dr. Dyson. He'd responded to the increasing numbers of young people showing up in the emergency room when it was too late by creating the Institute. This book is in part my call to action to the broader health crisis in urban communities.

For five years after my departure from the Institute, I worked under contract at a hospital in central New Jersey and another in Pennsylvania. The commute was exhausting, and I was grateful to return to the Newark area in 2012 to work on the emergency department staffs of two hospitals. In addition to my clinical work, I continue to reach out to young people through The Three Doctors Foundation. People often ask me if George, Rameck, and I are still friends—a question that always puzzles me. The bond that the three of us formed to pull one another up and out of poverty is lifelong, and we cherish the opportunities to get together to do our charity work and speaking engagements and, of course, to socialize. Rameck is a board-certified internist at University Medical Center of Princeton at Plainsboro and an assistant professor of medicine at Robert Wood Johnson Medical School, our alma mater. George recently got married and works as an assistant professor of clinical dentistry in the Department of Operative Dentistry at Columbia University College of Dental Medicine.

Since the publication of *The Pact,* the three of us have shared our story in a children's book, *We Beat the Streets*, and in a book about fatherhood and forgiveness, *The Bond: Three Young Men Learn to Forgive and Reconnect with Their Fathers.* By the time we began working on the last book, my father was too ill to participate, and he died before its completion. But I was grateful that

I had a chance to learn all I never knew about him and to grow a bit closer to him. In his final years, he trusted my advice and guidance in making sure he got the appropriate medical care for his prostate cancer and other health ailments. When he closed his eyes for good, I held no more bitterness toward him, just love.

My relationship with my father had for a long time left me somewhat fearful of becoming a father myself. What if I failed? I had friends who had grown up without fathers but became amazing fathers themselves by forging with their children the close bond they wished they'd shared with their own dads. My friends gave me hope that the same was possible for me. When my relationship with Melissa turned serious, we sometimes toyed with the idea of having a child together. I'd occasionally glance in the backseat of my car and wonder what it would be like to have a cooing baby strapped back there, relying on me to help him navigate the world. In October 2007, I was in San Francisco as part of a book tour when Melissa sent me a text message asking me to call her. As soon as I made it back to my hotel room, I sat at the desk and pulled out my phone.

"I have something to tell you," she said cheerfully. Being a doctor, I'd already noticed subtle changes in her body, and I was pretty sure I knew what she was about to say. Even so, I can't recall a happier moment in my life than when Melissa confirmed my suspicion: She was pregnant. I stared out the hotel window and allowed the news to sink in: *I was going to be a dad.*

My son, Jaxson Hayes Davis, was born on June 18, 2008. His life has brought even more clarity to my purpose, beyond the love, nurturing, and guidance that fatherhood requires. He makes it easier for me to believe that the safer, saner, healthier world that I envision for all children is possible if we all pitch in. For me, that has largely meant hands-on mentoring, just being there for kids like Malique. He was ten years old when his mother stood up in a

Newark bookstore and introduced him to George, Rameck, and me nearly a decade ago. The three of us have remained close to him ever since.

Malique recently completed his freshman year at Delaware State and is excited about pursuing a career in physical therapy. The two of us talk, text, and email regularly, but one day I was surprised to get a long, emotional letter from him. He seemed hardly able to believe that someone with no biological connection to him has cared enough to stick with him all these years, especially during the tough times. His genuine gratitude deeply moved me. I remember feeling the same sense of wonder and appreciation when I was in college and medical school and strangers who had no compelling reason to help me did. And they expected little in return, just that I do my best to succeed, and then that I remember what it took.

ACKNOWLEDGMENTS

Sampson Davis

The idea for this book came unexpectedly. One snowy winter evening many years ago, I was out to dinner with a friend and was sharing a medical story that had unfolded in the E.R. earlier that day. My phone rang, and I lost track of the story. When I got off the phone, my friend was still engaged in my story and demanded that I finish it. Right then, it occurred to me that others might have the same reaction, that I could use real-life drama to shine a spotlight on the health crisis in America's cities and show the potential consequences of bad decisions regarding personal health. We can learn through one another. It is my hope that this book creates ongoing dialogue and sparks a movement that pushes us all to take our fair piece of ownership in helping to heal our homes and communities.

First and foremost, I owe endless thanks to my patients and their families; their stories are all of our stories. To the families of the deceased, know that your loved ones live on through the words in this book, and although their names have been changed to protect their identities, their spirits are forever present to teach and heal.

This book was shaped with the tremendous support of my family, friends, mentors, co-workers, and patients from all walks of life. To you, I am eternally grateful; without you, life's meaning and purpose would be called into question. I attempt daily to walk in the light and direction of my Higher Power, and to God be the glory. I am ever striving to accomplish all that God has set forth as possible for me.

Thanks to my previous agent, Joann Davis, who introduced me to the agent for this book, Linda Loewenthal. Linda immediately saw the potential in my idea, shared my vision for it, and hit the ground running. Linda, I am forever grateful for your guidance throughout the entire process and your desire to help make this book all it could be. Lisa Frazier Page, who had worked with me as the writer of *The Pact,* was the obvious choice as my collaborator, and the timing for her was perfect. The two of us spent many hours talking on the phone, meeting in New Jersey and New York, and exchanging countless emails as we embraced the vision and worked to shape this project. Lisa, I remain overjoyed to have had the opportunity to reconnect and bring forth this project. As fate would have it, Spiegel & Grau, an imprint of the Random House Publishing Group, became the home for the book. Cindy Spiegel, senior vice president and publisher of the imprint, had been my editor on *The Pact.* Cindy, you are the best publisher and editor, hands down. Your brilliance shines through in all that you touch and again is masterfully displayed in this book. Thank you for your personal interest and involvement in this project. To the entire Spiegel & Grau team, especially Julie Grau, another brilliant editor and publisher, I am ecstatic to be a part of your literary reach.

To my mother, words alone can't express the magnitude and the depth of my love for you. Only you would take public transportation to Newark Beth Israel's emergency department and linger in the waiting room just to hear my name again and again over the intercom. Actions like this spoke louder than any words ever could about your pride in me. Melissa, from the pavement of Brooklyn our love grew, and our son, Jaxson, is a reflection of our bond. He is the perfect combination of the two of us. How blessed I am to have both of you in my world. To my deceased father and sister, Kenneth and Fellease Davis, I miss you and know you are smiling down from above. To my siblings—Kenny, Roselene, Andre, and Carlton—and my uncles, aunts, nieces, nephews, cousins, and family, we have been knocked down, but still together we stand. Love you all.

Carole Jackson, Mary Ann Jackson, and Frankie White, thank you for opening your home to me. My years spent on Hazelwood will be cherished forever. Newark Beth Israel Medical Center, University Hospital, and all of the hospitals where I have treated patients, I am forever thankful for having been part of dynamic crews of individuals who day in and day out give their all to the patients under their care.

Thanks to my circle of mentors, friends, and relatives, including Carla Dickson, Dr. Hsu, Reggie Brown, Camille, Sabu, Dax, Nnamdi, Will, Lawrence, Patrick, Maria, Al-Tereek, Hassan, Serron, Derrick Melba, Aunt Doretha, Darrell Terry, Dr. Dyson, Dr. Borenstein, Dr. Essien, Stephen Dunbar, Dr. Doctry, Anthony Davis, Thelma Davis, Trina, Lisa, Cynthia, Clarise, Renee, Valerie, Angelo, Edwin, Orlando, and Hashim. You have helped to shape my world and are a part of my everyday existence.

And then there are my two best friends, Dr. Rameck Hunt and Dr. George Jenkins, who with me make up The Three Doctors. Our pact is tighter than ever, and I'm thankful to travel this life with you both. To everyone who has embraced our message of health and education, and our pact of triumphing over inexplicable odds, I say "thank you." To the hundreds of high schools, colleges, graduate programs, special groups, community programs, and corporations that I have visited to share the story of The Three Doctors, thank you for embracing our message.

A handful of people have played a vital role in supporting me as part of The Three Doctors: Dr. Bill Cosby, Tavis Smiley, Sybil Wilkes, Tom Joyner, Cory Booker, Terrie Williams, Meredith Vieira, Joann Davis, Queen Latifah, Faith Evans, Marilyn Ducksworth, Susan Petersen Kennedy, Jake Morrissey, Geoff Kloske, Congressman Chaka Fattah, Dr. Steve Salvatore, Dr. Steve Adubato, Allan Houston, Stephen A. Smith, and Margaret Bernstein. I appreciate your unwavering support. To Windy White, the core group of volunteers for The Three Doctors Foundation, and our sponsors, your efforts are unparalleled; you keep the foundation alive and thriving. Special thanks to Jim Sinegal and Art Jackson for being there from day one. You may never know the lives you have touched.

Lastly, there are many others to whom I am forever indebted, those who have stood by me throughout this journey. I am lucky to call you friend, mentor, colleague, partner, brother, and sister. If I didn't name you specifically, please know that I hold you close in my heart and pray you understand what you mean to me.

As for my Brick City, we will continue to move forward. So much good exists in Newark, and I know we are capable of reaching new heights. Our people are eager to see and be part of a better today and tomorrow. Together we can soar.

Peace, love, and blessings,

Sampson

Lisa Frazier Page

I give all honor and praise to God for working through me to help this book come alive. My prayer is that this work will be received as intended: for good. Dr. Sampson Davis, thank you for never giving up on your vision to see this book in print and for choosing me as your literary partner. My respect for you has only grown as I've watched you up close and learned about the acts of kindness that you were too humble to share. To Linda, our literary agent, thanks, as always, for insisting on perfection, no matter how long it took. This project is better for it. Cindy, Julie, and the team at Spiegel & Grau, your collective talent notwithstanding, I most admire how deeply you care—about your books, your authors, and the messages we spread through you to the world. I'm so honored to be under your umbrella.

To my husband, Kevin, and our children, Enjoli, Danielle, Kevin Jr., and Kyle, I love you endlessly. Thank you for your understanding and patience while sharing me with this project for nearly four years. I was blessed with terrific parents, Clinton and Nettie Frazier, and parents-in-law, Richard and Miriam Page. I am strengthened daily by the love and prayers of our entire family, including Melissa and Ezron Moses, Clifford Frazier, April Bruns, Joseph and Joyce Richardson, Zina Page, Kolin and Geraldine Page, and the most supportive nieces, nephews, cousins, aunts, and uncles in the world. I couldn't have asked for a more generous employer, *The Washington Post,* which granted without hesitation the time off I needed to finish this book. I learned so much during my nearly seventeen years there as a writer and editor, and despite my departure this year, I still consider myself part of the family.

So many people have helped me along this journey that I can't call every name, but I have appreciated every kind word and deed. Nonetheless, I owe a special thanks to: Deadra and Stuart Courtney, Lavette Broussard, Tess Snipes, Cassandra and Frank Price, Veronica Smith, Cheryl Thompson, Donald Washington, Karima and Dion Haynes, Keith Woods, Milton Coleman, Vernon Loeb, Wil Haygood, DeNeen Brown, Carla Broyles, Lonnae O'Neal Parker, Avis Thomas-Lester, Monica Norton, Robert Pierre, Miranda Spivack, Erica Johnston, and my former A team of reporters, Tara Bahrampour, Michelle Boorstein, Pam Constable, Annie Gowen, Hamil Harris, and Carol Morello.

To my sisters of Delta Sigma Theta Sorority, Inc., particularly

Beta Gamma chapter alumnae and our own national president, Cynthia M. A. Butler-McIntyre, thanks for always having my back. Congratulations on one hundred years of service.

Finally, I wish to thank all of my teachers and mentors, especially the late Barbara Butler, and her husband, Eugene (Coach Butler), and Mrs. Ada Hannibal Green, who through the Spartanette Service Club opened the world to me when I was a sheltered teenager growing up in the piney woods of Bogalusa, Louisiana.

BIBLIOGRAPHY

"African Americans, Black Caribbeans, and Whites Differ in Depression Risk, Treatment." *National Institute of Mental Health.* National Institutes of Health, 5 Mar. 2007. Web. 18 July 2012. www.nimh.nih.gov/science-news/2007/african-americans-black-caribbeans-and-whites-differ-in-depression-risk-treatment.shtml.

"African Americans Disproportionately Affected by STDs." *Centers for Disease Control and Prevention.* Centers for Disease Control and Prevention, 01 June 2003. Web. 18 July 2012. www.cdc.gov/stdconference/2000/media/AfAmericans2000.htm.

"Asthma Facts and Figures." *Asthma Facts and Figures.* Asthma and Allergy Foundation of America, n.d. Web. 18 July 2012. www.aafa.org/display.cfm?id=8&sub=42.

Brady Campaign to Prevent Gun Violence : Race/Ethnicity. N.p., n.d. Web. 17 July 2012. www.bradycampaign.org/facts/gunviolence/factsethnicity.

Davis, Robert. "Many Lives Are Lost Across USA Because Emergency Services Fail." *USA Today,* 20 May 2005: A1. Print.

"Final Report of the Tuskegee Syphilis Study Legacy Committee." *University of Virginia Health System.* Claude Moore Health Sciences Library, 20 May 1996. Web. 18 July 2012. www.hsl.virginia.edu/historical/medical_history/bad_blood/report.cfm.

Flaherty, Mary Pat, Jenna Johnson, and Justin Jouvenal. "George Huguely Guilty of Second Degree Murder." *The Washington Post,* 22 Feb. 2012: A1. Print.

Hirsley, Michael. "Rev. Clements Leaves Behind Quite a Legacy." *Chicago Tribune.* Chicago Tribune, 23 June 1991. Web. 18 July 2012. http://articles

.chicagotribune.com/1991-06-23/news/9102250378_1_rev-george-clements
-legacy-campaigns.

"Homicide Trends in the U.S.: Trends by Race." *Bureau of Justice Statistics.*
U.S. Department of Justice, n.d. Web. 17 July 2012. http://bjs.ojp.usdoj.gov/
content/homicide/race.cfm.

Hu, Guoqing, Daniel Webster, and Susan P. Baker. "Hidden Homicide Increases
in the USA, 1999–2005." *Journal of Urban Health* 85.4 (2008): 597–606.
Print.

Jones, Charisse. "Violence Brings Club Crackdown." *USA Today* [Arlington],
4 Apr. 2007: A1. Print.

Kaegi, Louise. "What Color Is Your Pain." N.p., Summer 2004. Web. 18 July
2012.

Katz, Ralph V., S. Steven Kegeles, Nancy R. Kressin, B. Lee Green, Min Qi
Wang, Sherman A. James, Stefanie Luise Russell, and Cristina Claudio.
"The Tuskegee Legacy Project: Willingness of Minorities to Participate in
Biomedical Research." *Journal of Health Care for the Poor and Under-
served* 17.4 (2006): 698-715. Print.

Langley, Marty. "Black Homicide Victimization in the United States: An Analysis
of 2007 Homicide Data." *Violence Policy Center.* Jan. 2010. Web. 17 July
2012. www.vpc.org/studies/blackhomicide10.pdf.

McNeil Jr., Donald G. "U.S. Apologizes for Syphilis Tests in Guatemala." *The
New York Times,* 1 Oct. 2010: A1. Print.

"NACAC | How to Adopt." *NACAC | How to Adopt.* North American Coun-
cil on Adoptable Children, n.d. Web. 18 July 2012. www.nacac.org/
howtoadopt/adoptiontypes.html.

"Nation's Leading Experts Confirm College Dating Violence Is a Much Larger
Problem Than Anyone Realizes." *Love Is Not Abuse: Home.* Liz Claiborne
Inc., 14 Sept. 2011. Web. 12 Apr. 2012. www.loveisnotabuse.com/.

Nolin, Robert. "Body Count Mounts with South Florida Nightclub Killings on
the Rise." *Sun-Sentinel* [Fort Lauderdale], 27 Feb. 2012: A1. Print.

Paulozzi, Leonard J., Christopher M. Jones, Karin A. Mack, Rose A. Rudd.
"Vital Signs: Overdoses of Prescription Opioid Pain Relievers—United
States, 1999–2008." *Morbidity and Mortality Weekly Report.* Centers for
Disease Control and Prevention, 2011. Web. 4 Nov. 2011. www.cdc.gov/
mmwr/preview/mmwrhtml/mm6043a4.htm.

"Protect Children, Not Guns 2009." *Children's Defense Fund.* Children's
Defense Fund, 16 Sept. 2009. Web. 17 July 2012. www.childrensdefense

.org/child-research-data-publications/data/protect-children-not-guns -report-2009.html.

"Results from the 2010 National Survey on Drug Use and Health: Summary of National Findings." *Substance Abuse and Mental Health Services Administration*. U.S. Department of Health and Human Services, Sept. 2011. Web. 17 July 2012. www.samhsa.gov/data/nsduh/2k10NSDUH/2k10Results.pdf.

Sexually Transmitted Disease Surveillance 2010. Rep. Atlanta: Centers for Disease Control and Prevention, 2011. Print.

Tang, Ning, John Stein, Renee Y. Hsia, Judith Maselli, and Ralph Gonzales. "Trends and Characteristics of U.S. Emergency Department Visits, 1997–2007." *PubMed Central*. National Institutes of Health, 11 Aug. 2010. Web. 18 July 2012. www.ncbi.nlm.nih.gov/pmc/articles/PMC3123697/.

Vandivere, Sharon, Karen Malm, and Laura Radel. *Adoption USA: A Chartbook Based on the 2007 National Survey of Adoptive Parents*. Washington, D.C.: U.S. Department of Health and Human Services, Office of the Assistant Secretary for Planning and Evaluation, 2009. Print.

ABOUT THE AUTHORS

Dr. Sampson Davis

Sampson Davis was born and raised in Newark, New Jersey. He received his bachelor's degree from Seton Hall University and his medical degree from Robert Wood Johnson Medical School, and he completed his residency in emergency medicine at the same hospital where he was born, Newark Beth Israel Medical Center.

Dr. Davis is a board-certified emergency medicine physician and co-author of *The New York Times* bestsellers *The Pact*, *We Beat the Street,* and *The Bond*. The youngest physician to receive the National Medical Association's highest honor, the Scroll of Merit, he has also received *Essence* and BET humanitarian awards, and was named by *Essence* as one of the forty most inspirational African Americans. He is a founder of The Three Doctors Foundation, focusing on health, education, leadership, and mentoring. Dr. Davis has appeared in various print publications and on numerous national television and radio news and talk shows, including *Oprah,* the *Today* show, and *The View,* and has served as a medical correspondent for CNN and *The Tom Joyner Morning Show*. He practices emergency medicine in New Jersey.

Dr. Davis is available for select readings and lectures. To inquire about a possible appearance, please email *drsampsondavis@gmail.com*.

www.drsampsondavis.com

Lisa Frazier Page

LISA FRAZIER PAGE is a writer living in the New Orleans area. She worked for nearly seventeen years as a reporter and editor at *The Washington Post* and for a decade as a writer at *The Times-Picayune* newspaper in New Orleans.

She was a co-writer of the *New York Times* bestseller *The Pact: Three Young Men Make a Promise and Fulfill a Dream,* published in 2002. She also collaborated with Carlotta Walls LaNier, the youngest member of the Little Rock Nine, on LaNier's 2009 memoir, *A Mighty Long Way: My Journey to Justice at Little Rock Central High School.*

Page holds a master's degree from Northwestern University's Medill School of Journalism, and a bachelor's from Dillard University in New Orleans. She and her husband, Kevin, have four children.

ABOUT THE TYPE

This book was set in Sabon, a typeface designed by the well-known German typographer Jan Tschichold (1902–74). Sabon's design is based upon the original letter forms of Claude Garamond and was created specifically to be used for three sources: foundry type for hand composition, Linotype, and Monotype. Tschichold named his typeface for the famous Frankfurt typefounder Jacques Sabon, who died in 1580.